The Hermit of Far End

Margaret Pedler

Contents

THE HERMIT OF FAR END

BY

Margaret Pedler

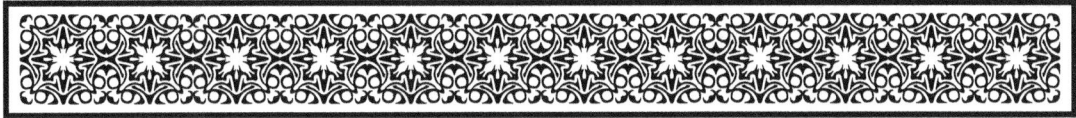

PROLOGUE

It was very quiet within the little room perched high up under the roof of Wallater's Buildings. Even the glowing logs in the grate burned tranquilly, without any of those brisk cracklings and sputterings which make such cheerful company of a fire, while the distant roar of London's traffic came murmuringly, dulled to a gentle monotone by the honeycomb of narrow side streets that intervened between the gaunt, red-brick Buildings and the bustling highways of the city.

It seemed almost as though the little room were waiting for something--some one, just as the woman seated in the low chair at the hearthside was waiting.

She sat very still, looking towards the door, her folded hands lying quietly on her knees in an attitude of patient expectancy. It was as if, although she found the waiting long and wearisome, she were yet quite sure she would not have to wait in vain.

Once she bent forward and touched the little finger of her left hand, which bore, at its base, a slight circular depression such as comes from the constant wearing of a ring. She rubbed it softly with the forefinger of the other hand.

"He will come," she muttered. "He promised he would come if ever I sent the little pearl ring."

Then she leaned back once more, resuming her former attitude of patient waiting, and the insistent silence, momentarily broken by her movement, settled down again upon the room.

Presently the long rays of the westering sun crept round the edge of some projecting eaves and, slanting in suddenly through the window, rested upon the quiet figure in the chair.

Even in their clear, revealing light it would have been difficult to decide the woman's age, so worn and lined was the mask-like face outlined against the shabby cushion. She looked forty, yet there was something still girlish in the pose of her black-clad figure which seemed to suggest a shorter tale of years. Raven dark hair, lustreless and dull, framed a pale, emaciated face from which ill-health had stripped almost all that had once been beautiful. Only the immense dark eyes, feverishly bright beneath the sunken temples, and the still lovely line from jaw to pointed chin, remained unmarred, their beauty mocked by the pinched nostrils and drawn mouth, and by the scraggy, almost fleshless throat.

It might have been the face of a dead woman, so still, so waxen was it, were it not for the eager brilliance of the eyes. In them, fixed watchfully upon the closed door, was concentrated the whole vitality of the failing body.

Beyond that door, flight upon flight of some steps dropped seemingly endlessly one below the other, leading at last to a cement-floored vestibule, cheerless and uninviting, which opened on to the street.

Perhaps there was no particular reason why the vestibule should have been other than it was, seeing that Wallater's Buildings had not been designed for the habitual loiterer. For such as he there remains always the "luxurious entrance-hall" of hotel advertisement.

As far as the inhabitants of "Wallater's" were concerned, they clattered over the cement flooring of the vestibule in the mornings, on their way to work, without pausing to cast an eye of criticism upon its general aspect of uncomeliness, and dragged tired feet across it in an evening with no other thought but that of how many weary steps there were to climb before the room which served as "home" should be attained.

But to the well-dressed, middle-aged man who now paused, half in doubt, on the threshold of the Buildings, the sordid-looking vestibule, with its bare floor and drab-coloured walls, presented an epitome of desolation.

His keen blue eyes, in one of which was stuck a monocle attached to a broad black ribbon, rested appraisingly upon the ascending spiral of the stone stairway that vanished into the gloomy upper reaches of the Building.

Against this chill background there suddenly took shape in his mind the picture of a spacious room, fragrant with the scent of roses--a room full of mellow tints of brown and gold, athwart which the afternoon sunlight lingered tenderly, picking out here the limpid blue of a bit of old Chinese "blue-and-white," there the warm gleam of polished copper, or here again the bizarre, gem-encrusted image of an Eastern god. All that was rare and beautiful had gone to the making of the room, and rarer and more beautiful than all, in the eyes of the man whose memory now recalled it, had been the woman to whom it had belonged, whose loveliness had glowed within it like a jewel in a rich setting.

With a mental jolt his thoughts came back to the present, to the bare, commonplace ugliness of Wallater's Buildings.

"My God!" he muttered. "Pauline--here!"

Then with swift steps he began the ascent of the stone steps, gradually slackening in pace until, when he reached the summit and stood facing that door behind which a woman watched and waited, he had perforce to pause to regain his breath, whilst certain twinges in his right knee reminded him that he was no longer as young as he had been.

In answer to his knock a low voice bade him enter, and a minute later he was standing in the quiet little room, his eyes gazing levelly into the feverish dark ones of the woman who had risen at his entrance.

"So!" she said, while an odd smile twisted her bloodless lips. "You have come, after all. Sometimes--I began to doubt if you would. It is days--an eternity since I sent for you."

"I have been away," he replied simply. "And my mail was not forwarded. I came directly I received the ring--at once, as I told you I should."

"Well, sit down and let us talk"--impatiently--"it doesn't matter--nothing matters since you have come in time."

"In time? What do you mean? In time for what? Pauline, tell me"--advancing a step--"tell me, in God's Name, what are you doing in this place?" He glanced significantly round the shabby room with its threadbare carpet and distempered walls.

"I'm living here--"

"*Living here? You?*"

"Yes. Why not? Soon"--indifferently--"I shall be dying here. It is, at least, as good a place to die in as any other."

"Dying?" The man's pleasant baritone voice suddenly shook. "Dying? Oh, no, no! You've been ill--I can see that--but with care and good nursing--"

"Don't deceive yourself, my friend," she interrupted him remorselessly. "See, come to the window. Now look at me--and then don't talk any more twaddle about care and good nursing!"

She had drawn him towards the window, till they were standing together in the full blaze of the setting sun. Then she turned and faced him--a gaunt wreck of splendid womanhood, her fingers working nervously, whilst her too brilliant eyes, burning in their grey, sunken, sockets, searched his face curiously.

"You've worn better than I have," she observed at last, breaking the silence with a short laugh, "you must be--let me see--fifty. While I'm barely thirty-one--and I look forty--and the rest."

Suddenly he reached out and gathered her thin, restless hands into his, holding them in a kind, firm clasp.

"Oh, my dear!" he said sadly. "Is there nothing I can do?"

"Yes," she answered steadily. "There is. And it's to ask you if you will do it that I sent for you. Do you suppose"--she swallowed, battling with the tremor in her voice--"that I *wanted* you to see me--as I am now? It was months--months before I could bring myself to send you the little pearl ring."

He stooped and kissed one of the hands he held.

"Dear, foolish woman! You would always be--just Pauline--to me."

Her eyes softened suddenly.

"So you never married, after all?"

He straightened his shoulders, meeting her glance squarely--almost sternly.

"Did you imagine that I should?" he asked quietly.

"No, no, I suppose not." She looked away. "What a mess I made of things, didn't I? However, it's all past now; the game's nearly over, thank Heaven! Life, since that day"--the eyes of the man and woman met again in swift understanding--"has been one long hell."

"He--the man you married--"

"Made that hell. I left him after six years of it, taking the child with me."

"The child?" A curious expression came into his eyes, resentful, yet tinged at the same time with an oddly tender interest. "Was there a child?"

"Yes--I have a little daughter."

"And did your husband never trace you?" he asked, after a pause.

"He never tried to"--grimly. "Afterwards--well, it was downhill all the way. I didn't know how to work, and by that time I had learned my health was going. Since then, I've lived on the proceeds of the pawnshop--I had my jewels, you know--and on the odd bits of money I could scrape together by taking in sewing."

A groan burst from the man's dry lips.

"Oh, my God!" he cried. "Pauline, Pauline, it was cruel of you to keep me in ignorance! I could at least have helped."

She shook her head.

"I couldn't take--*your* money," she said quietly. "I was too proud for that. But, dear friend"--as she saw him wince--"I'm not proud any longer. I think Death very soon shows us how little--pride--matters; it falls into its right perspective when one is nearing the end of things. I'm so little proud now that I've sent for you to ask your help."

"Anything--anything!" he said eagerly.

"It's rather a big thing that I'm going to ask, I'm afraid. I want you," she spoke slowly, as though to focus his attention, "to take care of my child--when I am gone."

He stared at her doubtfully.

"But her father? Will he consent?" he asked.

"He is dead. I received the news of his death six months ago. There is no one--no one who has any claim upon her. And no one upon whom she has any claim, poor little atom!"--smiling rather bitterly. "Ah! Don't deny me!"--her thin, eager hands clung to his--"don't deny me--say that you'll take her!"

"Deny you? But, of course I shan't deny you. I'm only thankful that you have turned to me at last--that you have not quite forgotten!"

"Forgotten?" Her voice vibrated. "Believe me or not, as you will, there has never been a day for nine long years when I have not remembered--never a night when I have not prayed God to bless you----" She broke off, her mouth working uncontrollably.

Very quietly, very tenderly, he drew her into his arms. There was no passion in the caress--for was it not eventide, and the lengthening shadows of night already fallen across her path?--but there was infinite love, and forgiveness, and understanding. . . .

"And now, may I see her--the little daughter?"

The twilight had gathered about them during that quiet hour of reunion, wherein old hurts had been healed, old sins forgiven, and now at last they had come back together out of the past to the recognition of all that yet remained to do.

There came a sound of running footsteps on the stairs outside--light, eager steps, buoyant with youth, that evidently found no hardship in the long ascent from the street level.

"Hark!" The woman paused, her head a little turned to listen. "Here she comes. No one else on this floor"--with a whimsical smile--"could take the last flight of those awful stairs at a run."

The door flew open, and the man received an impressionist picture of which the salient features were a mop of black hair, a scarlet jersey, and a pair of abnormally long black legs.

Then the door closed with a bang, and the blur of black and scarlet resolved itself into a thin, eager-faced child of eight, who paused irresolutely upon perceiving a stranger in the room.

"Come here, kiddy," the woman held out her hand. "This"--and her eyes sought those of the man as though beseeching confirmation--"is your uncle."

The child advanced and shook hands politely, then stood still, staring at this unexpectedly acquired relative.

Her sharp-pointed face was so thin and small that her eyes, beneath their straight, dark brows, seemed to be enormous--black, sombre eyes, having no kinship with the intense, opaque brown so frequently miscalled black, but suggestive of the vibrating darkness of night itself.

Instinctively the man's glance wandered to the face of the child's mother.

"You think her like me?" she hazarded.

"She is very like you," he assented gravely.

A wry smile wrung her mouth.

"Let us hope that the likeness is only skin-deep, then!" she said bitterly. "I don't want her life to be--as mine has been."

"If," he said gently, "if you will trust her to me, Pauline, I swear to you that I will do all in my power to save her from--what you've suffered."

The woman shrugged her shoulders.

"It's all a matter of character," she said nonchalantly.

"Yes," he agreed simply. Then he turned to the child, who was standing a little distance away from him, eyeing him distrustfully. "What do you say, child! You wouldn't be afraid to come and live with me, would you?"

"I am never afraid of people," she answered promptly. "Except the man who comes for the rent; he is fat, and red, and a beast. But I'd rather go on living with Mumsy, thank you--Uncle." The designation came after a brief hesitation. "You see," she added politely, as though fearful that she might have hurt his feelings, "we've always lived together." She flung a glance of almost passionate adoration at her mother, who turned towards the man, smiling a little wistfully.

"You see how it is with her?" she said. "She lives by her affections--conversely from her mother, her heart rules her head. You will be gentle with her, won't you, when the wrench comes?"

"My dear," he said, taking her hand in his and speaking with the quiet solemnity of a man who vows himself before some holy altar, "I shall never forget that she is your child--the child of the woman I love."

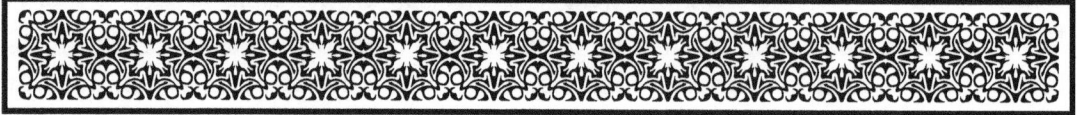

CHAPTER I
A MORNING ADVENTURE

The dewy softness of early morning still hung about the woods, veiling their autumn tints in broken, drifting swathes of pearly mist, while towards the east, where the rising sun pushed long, dim fingers of light into the murky greyness of the sky, a tremulous golden haze grew and deepened.

Little, delicate twitterings vibrated on the air--the sleepy chirrup of awakening birds, the rustle of a fallen leaf beneath the pad of some belated cat stealing back to the domestic hearth, the stir of a rabbit in its burrow.

Presently these sank into insignificance beside a more definite sound--the crackle of dry leaves and the snapping of twigs beneath a heavier footfall than that of any marauding Tom, and through a clearing in the woods slouched the figure of a man, gun on shoulder, the secret of his bulging side-pockets betrayed by the protruding tail feathers of a cock-pheasant.

He was not an attractive specimen of mankind. Beneath the peaked cap, crammed well down on to his head, gleamed a pair of surly, watchful eyes, and, beneath these again, the unshaven, brutal, out-thrust jaw offered little promise of better things.

Nor did his appearance in any way belie his reputation, which was unsavory in the extreme. Indeed, if report spoke truly, "Black Brady," as he was commonly called, had on one occasion only escaped the gallows thanks to the evidence of a village girl--one who had loved him recklessly, to her own undoing. Every one had believed her evidence to be false, but, as she had stuck to what she said through thick and thin, and as no amount of cross-examination had been able to shake her, Brady had contrived to slip through the hands of the police.

Conceiving, however, that, after this episode, the air of his native place might prove somewhat insalubrious for a time, he had migrated thence to Fallowdene, establishing himself in a cottage on the outskirts of the village and finding the major portion of his sustenance by skillfully poaching the preserves of the principal land-owners of the surrounding district.

On this particular morning he was well content with his night's work. He had raided the covers of one Patrick Lovell, the owner of Barrow Court, who, although himself a confirmed invalid and debarred from all manner of sport, employed two or three objectionably lynx-eyed keepers to safeguard his preserves for the benefit of his heirs and assigns.

No covers were better stocked than those of Barrow Court, but Brady rarely risked replenishing his larder from them, owing to the extreme wideawakeness of the head gamekeeper. It was therefore not without a warm glow of satisfaction about the region of his heart that he made his way homeward through the early morning, reflecting on the ease with which last night's marauding expedition had been conducted. He even pursed his lips together and whistled softly--a low, flute-like sound that might almost have been mistaken for the note of a blackbird.

But it is unwise to whistle before you are out of the wood, and Brady's triumph was short-lived. Swift as a shadow, a lithe figure darted out from among the trees and planted itself directly in his path.

With equal swiftness, Brady brought his gunstock to his shoulder. Then he hesitated, finger on trigger, for the lion in his path was no burly gamekeeper, as, for the first moment, he had supposed. It was a woman who faced him--a mere girl of twenty, whose slender figure looked somehow boyish in its knitted sports coat and very short, workmanlike skirt. The suggestion of boyishness was emphasized by her attitude, as she stood squarely planted in front of Black Brady, her hands thrust deep into her pockets, her straight young back very flat, and her head a little tilted, so that her eyes might search the surly face beneath the peaked cap.

They were arresting eyes--amazingly dark, "like two patches o' the sky be night," as Brady described them long afterwards to a crony of his, and they gazed up at the astonished poacher from a small, sharply angled face, as delicately cut as a cameo.

"Put that gun down!" commanded an imperious young voice, a voice that held something indescribably sweet and thrilling in its vibrant quality. "What are you doing in these woods?"

Brady, recovering from his first surprise, lowered his gun, but answered truculently--

"Never you mind what I'm doin'."

The girl pointed significantly to his distended pockets.

"I don't need to ask. Empty out your pockets and take yourself off. Do you hear?" she added sharply, as the man made no movement to obey.

"I shan't do nothin' o' the sort," he growled. "You go your ways and leave me to go mine--or it'll be the worse for 'ee." He raised his gun threateningly.

The girl smiled.

"I'm not in the least afraid of that gun," she said tranquilly. "But you are afraid to use it," she added.

"Am I?" He wheeled suddenly, and, on the instant, a deafening report shattered the quiet of the woods. Then the smoke drifted slowly aside, revealing the man and the girl face to face once more.

But although she still stood her ground, dark shadows had suddenly painted themselves beneath her eyes, and the slight young breast beneath the jaunty sports coat rose and fell unevenly. Within the shelter of her coat-pockets her hands were clenched tightly.

"That was a waste of a good cartridge," she observed quietly. "You only fired in the air."

Black Brady glared at her.

"If I'd liked, I could 'ave killed 'ee as easy as knockin' a bird off a bough," he said sullenly.

"You could," she agreed. "And then I should have been dead and you would have been waiting for a hanging. Of the two, I think my position would have been the more comfortable."

A look of unwilling admiration spread itself slowly over the man's face.

"You be a cool 'and, and no mistake," he acknowledged. "I thought to frighten you off by firin'."

The girl nodded.

"Well, as you haven't, suppose you allow that I've won and that it's up to me to dictate terms. If my uncle were to see you--"

"I'm not comin' up to the house--don't you think it, win or no win," broke in Brady hastily.

The girl regarded him judicially.

"I don't think we particularly want you up at the house," she remarked. "If you'll do as I say--empty your pockets--you may go."

The man reluctantly made as though to obey, but even while he hesitated, he saw the girl's eyes suddenly look past him, over his shoulder, and, turning suspiciously, he swung straight into the brawny grip of the head keeper, who, hearing a shot fired, had deserted his breakfast and hurried in the direction of the sound and now came up close behind him.

"Caught this time, Brady, my man," chuckled the keeper triumphantly. "It's gaol for you this journey, as sure's my name's Clegg. Has the fellow been annoying you, Miss Sara?" he added, touching his hat respectfully as he turned towards the girl, whilst with his other hand he still retained his grip of Brady's arm.

She laughed as though suddenly amused.

"Nothing to speak of, Clegg," she replied. "And I'm afraid you mustn't send him to prison this time. I told him if he would empty his pockets he might go. That still holds good," she added, looking towards Brady, who flashed her a quick look of gratitude from beneath his heavy brows and proceeded to turn out the contents of his pockets with commendable celerity.

But the keeper protested against the idea of releasing his prisoner.

"It's a fair cop, miss," he urged entreatingly.

"Can't help it, Clegg. I promised. So you must let him go."

The man obeyed with obvious reluctance. Then, when Brady had hastened to make himself scarce, he turned and scrutinized the girl curiously.

"You all right, Miss Sara? Shall I see you up to the house?"

"No, thanks, Clegg," she said. "I'm--I'm quite all right. You can go back to your breakfast."

"Very good, miss." He touched his hat and plunged back again into the woods.

The girl stood still, looking after him. She was rather white, but she remained very erect and taut until the keeper had disappeared from view. Then the tense rigidity of her figure slackened, as a stretched wire slackens when the pull on it suddenly ceases, and she leaned helpless against the trunk of a tree, limp and shaking, every fine-strung nerve ajar with the strain of her recent encounter with Black Brady. As she felt her knees giving way weakly beneath her, a dogged little smile twisted her lips.

"You are a cool 'and, and no mistake," she whispered shakily, an ironical gleam flickering in her eyes.

She propped herself up against the friendly tree, and, after a few minutes, the quick throbbing of her heard steadied down and the colour began to steal back into her lips. At length she stooped, and, picking up her hat, which had fallen off and lay on the ground at her feet, she proceeded to make her way through the woods in the direction of the house.

Barrow Court, as the name implied, was situated on the brow of a hill, sheltered from the north and easterly winds by a thick belt of pines which half-encircled it, for ever murmuring and whispering together as pine-trees will.

To Sara Tennant, the soft, sibilant noise was a beloved and familiar sound. From the first moment when, as a child, she had come to live at Barrow, the insistent murmur of the pines had held an extraordinary fascination for her. That, and their pungent scent, seemed to be interwoven with her whole life there, like the thread of some single colour that persists throughout the length of a woven fabric.

She had been desperately miserable and lonely at the time of her advent at the Court; and all through the long, wakeful vigil of her first night, it had seemed to her vivid, childish imagination as though the big, swaying trees, bleakly etched against the moonlit sky, had understood her desolation and had whispered and crooned consolingly outside her window. Since then, she had learned that the voice of the pines, like the voice of the sea, is always pitched in a key that responds to the mood of the listener. If you chance to be glad, then the pines will whisper of sunshine and summer, little love idylls that one tree tells to another, but if your heart is heavy within you, you will hear only a dirge in the hush of their waving tops.

As Sara emerged from the shelter of the woods, her eyes instinctively sought the great belt of trees that crowned the opposite hill, with the grey bulk of the house standing out in sharp relief against their eternal green. A little smile of pure pleasure flitted across her face; to her there was something lovable and rather charming about the very architectural inconsistencies which prevented Barrow Court from being, in any sense of the word, a show place.

The central portion of the house, was comparatively modern, built of stone in solid Georgian fashion, but quaintly flanked at either end by a massive, mediaeval tower, survival of the good old days when the Lovells of Fallowdene had held their own against all comers, not even excepting, in the case of one Roderic, his liege lord and master the King, the latter having conceived a not entirely unprovoked desire to deprive him of his lands and liberty--a desire destined, however, to be frustrated by the solid masonry of Barrow.

A flagged terrace ran the whole length of the long, two-storied house, broadening out into wide wings at the base of either tower, and, below the terrace, green, shaven lawns, dotted with old yew, sloped down to the edge of a natural lake which lay in the hollow of the valley, gleaming like a sheet of silver in the morning sunlight.

Prim walks, bordered by high box hedges, intersected the carefully tended gardens, and along one of these Sara took her way, quickening her steps to a run as the booming summons of a gong suddenly reverberated on the air.

She reached the house, flushed and a little breathless, and, tossing aside her hat as she sped through the big, oak-beamed hall, hurried into a pleasant, sunshiny room, where a couple of menservants were moving quietly about, putting the finishing touches to the breakfast table.

An invalid's wheeled chair stood close to the open window, and in it, with a rug tucked about his knees, was seated an elderly man of some sixty-two or three years of age. He was leaning forward, giving animated instructions to a gardener who listened attentively from the terrace outside, and his alert, eager, manner contrasted oddly with the helplessness of limb indicated by the necessity for the wheeled chair.

"That's all, Digby," he said briskly. "I'll go through the hot-houses myself some time to-day."

As he spoke, he signed to one of the footmen in the room to close the window, and then propelled his chair with amazing rapidity to the table.

The instant and careful attention accorded to his commands by both gardener and servant was characteristic of every one in Patrick Lovell's employment. Although he had been a more or less helpless invalid for seven years, he had never lost his grip of things. He was exactly as much master of Barrow Court, the dominant factor there, as he had been in the good times that were gone, when no day's shooting had been too long for him, no run with hounds too fast.

He sat very erect in his wheeled chair, a handsome, well-groomed old aristocrat. Clean-shaven, except for a short, carefully trimmed moustache, grizzled like his hair, his skin exhibited the waxen pallor which so often accompanies chronic ill-health, and his face was furrowed by deep lines, making him look older than his sixty-odd years. His vivid blue eyes were extraordinarily keen and penetrating; possibly they, and the determined, squarish jaw, were answerable for that unquestioning obedience which was invariably accorded him.

"Good-morning, uncle mine!" Sara bent to kiss him as the door closed quietly behind the retreating servants.

Patrick Lovell screwed his monocle into his eye and regarded her dispassionately.

"You look somewhat ruffled," he observed, "both literally and figuratively."

She laughed, putting up a careless hand to brush back the heavy tress of dark hair that had fallen forward over her forehead.

"I've had an adventure," she answered, and proceeded to recount her experience with Black Brady. When she reached the point where the man had fired off his gun, Patrick interrupted explosively.

"The infernal scoundrel! That fellow will dangle at the end of a rope one of these days--and deserve it, too. He's a murderous ruffian--a menace to the countryside."

"He only fired into the air--to frighten me," explained Sara.

Her uncle looked at her curiously.

"And did he succeed?" he asked.

She bestowed a little grin of understanding upon him.

"He did," she averred gravely. Then, as Patrick's bushy eyebrows came together in a bristling frown, she added: "But he remained in ignorance of the fact."

The frown was replaced by a twinkle.

"That's all right, then," came the contented answer.

"All the same, I really *was* frightened," she persisted. "It gave me quite a nasty turn, as the servants say. I don't think"--meditatively--"that I enjoy being shot at. Am I a funk, my uncle?"

"No, my niece"--with some amusement. "On the contrary, I should define the highest type of courage as self-control in the presence of danger--not necessarily absence of fear. The latter is really no more credit to you than eating your dinner when you're hungry."

"Mine, then, I perceive to be the highest type of courage," chuckled Sara. "It's a comforting reflection."

It was, when propounded by Patrick Lovell, to whom physical fear was an unknown quantity. Had he lived in the days of the Terror, he would assuredly have taken his way to the guillotine with the same gay, debonair courage which enabled the nobles of France to throw down their cards and go to the scaffold with a smiling promise to the other players that they would continue their interrupted game in the next world.

And when Sara had come to live with Patrick, a dozen years ago, he had rigorously inculcated in her youthful mind a contempt for every form of cowardice, moral and physical.

It had not been all plain sailing, for Sara was a highly strung child, with the vivid imagination that is the primary cause of so much that is carelessly designated cowardice. But Patrick had been very wise in his methods. He had never rebuked her for lack of courage; he had simply taken it for granted that she would keep her grip of herself.

Sara's thoughts slid back to an incident which had occurred during their early days together. She had been very much alarmed by the appearance of a huge mastiff who was permitted the run of the house, and her uncle, noticing her shrinking avoidance of the rather formidable looking beast, had composedly bidden her take him to the stables and chain him up. For an instant the child had hesitated. Then, something in the man's quiet confidence that she would obey had made its claim on her childish pride, and, although white to the lips, she had walked straight up to the great creature, hooked her small fingers into his collar, and marched him off to his kennel.

Courage under physical pain she had learned from seeing Patrick contend with his own infirmity. He suffered intensely at times, but neither groan nor word of complaint was ever allowed to escape his set lips. Only Sara would see, after what he described as "one of my damn bad days, m'dear," new lines added to the deepening network that had so aged his appearance lately.

At these times she herself endured agonies of reflex suffering and apprehension, since her attachment to Patrick Lovell was the moving factor of her existence. Other girls had parents, brothers and sisters, and still more distant relatives upon whom their capacity for loving might severally expend itself. Sara had none of these, and the whole devotion of her intensely ardent nature lavished itself upon the man whom she called uncle.

Their mutual attitude was something more than the accepted relationship implied. They were friends--these two--intimate friends, comrades on an equal footing, respecting each other's reserves and staunchly loyal to one another. Perhaps this was accounted for in a measure by the very fact that they were united by no actual bond of blood. That Sara was Patrick's niece by adoption was all the explanation of her presence at Barrow Court that he had ever vouchsafed to the world in general, and it practically amounted to the sum total of Sara's own knowledge of the matter.

Hers had been a life of few relationships. She had no recollection of any one who had ever stood towards her in the position of a father, and though she realized that the one-time existence of such a personage must be assumed, she had never felt much curiosity concerning him.

The horizon of her earliest childhood had held but one figure, that of an adored mother, and "home" had been represented by a couple of meager rooms at the top of a big warren of a place known as Wallater's Buildings, tenanted principally by families of the artisan class.

Thus debarred by circumstances from the companionship of other children, Sara's whole affections had centred round her mother, and she had never forgotten the sheer, desolating anguish of that moment when the dreadful, unresponsive silence of the sheeted figure, lying in the shabby little bedroom they had shared together, brought home to her the significance of death.

She had not cried, as most children of eight would have done, but she had suffered in a kind of frozen silence, incapable of any outward expression of grief.

"Unfeelin', I call it!" declared the woman who lived on the same floor as the Tennants, and who had attended at the doctor's behest, to a friend and neighbour who was occupied in boiling a kettle over a gas-ring. "Must be a cold-'earted child as can see 'er own mother lyin' dead without so much as a tear." She sniffed. "'Aven't you got that cup o' tea ready yet? I can allus drink a cup o' tea after a layin'-out."

Sara had watched the two women drinking their tea with brooding eyes, her small breast heaving with the intensity of her resentment. Without being in any way able to define her emotions, she felt that there was something horrible in their frank enjoyment of the steaming liquid, gulped down to the cheerful accompaniment of a running stream of intimate gossip, while all the time that quiet figure lay on the narrow bed--motionless, silent, wrapped in the strange and immense aloofness of the dead.

Presently one of the women poured out a third cup of tea and pushed it towards the child, slopping in the thin, bluish-looking milk with a generous hand.

"'Ave a cup, child. It's as good a drop o' tea as ever I tasted."

For a moment Sara stared at her speechlessly; then, with a sudden passionate gesture, she swept the cup on to the floor.

The clash of breaking china seemed to ring through the chamber of death, the women's voices rose shrilly in reproof, and Sara, fleeing into the adjoining room, cast herself face downwards upon the floor, horror-stricken. It was not the raucous anger of the women which she heeded; that passed her by. But she had outraged some fine, instinctive sense by reverence that lay deep within her own small soul.

Still she did not cry. Only, as she lay on the ground with her face hidden, she kept repeating in a tense whisper--

"You know I didn't mean it, God! You know I didn't mean it!"

It was then that Patrick Lovell had appeared, coming in response to she knew not what summons, and had taken her away with him. And the tendrils of her affection, wrenched from their accustomed hold, had twined themselves about this grey-haired, blue-eyed man, set so apart by every ***soigné*** detail of his person from the shabby, slip-shod world which Sara had known, but who yet stood beside the bed on which her mother lay, with a wrung mouth beneath his clipped moustache and a mist of tears dimming his keen eyes.

Sara had loved him for those tears.

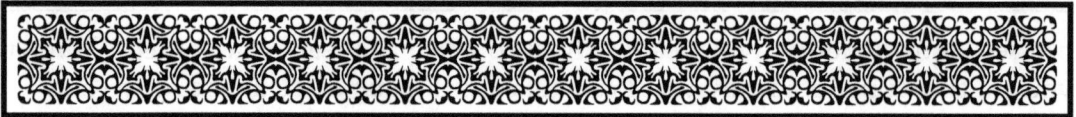

CHAPTER II
THE PASSING OF PATRICK LOVELL

Autumn had given place to winter, and a bitter northeast wind was tearing through the pines, shrieking, as it fled, like the cry of a lost soul. The eerie sound of it served in some indefinable way to emphasise the cosy warmth and security of the room where Sara and her uncle were sitting, their chairs drawn close up to the log fire which burned on the wide, old-fashioned hearth.

Sara was engrossed in a book, her head bent low above its pages, unconscious of the keen blue eyes that had been regarding her reflectively for some minutes.

With the passage of the last two months, Patrick's face seemed to have grown more waxen, worn a little finer, and now, as he sat quietly watching the slender figure on the opposite side of the hearth, it wore a curious, inscrutable expression, as though he were mentally balancing the pros and cons of some knotty point.

At last he apparently came to a decision, for he laid aside the newspaper he had been reading a few moments before, muttering half audibly:

"Must take your fences as you come to 'em."

Sara looked up abstractedly.

"Did you say anything?" she asked doubtfully.

Patrick gave his shoulders a grim shake.

"I'm going to," he replied. "It's something that must be said, and, as I've never been in favour of postponing a thing just because its disagreeable, we may as well get it over."

He had focused Sara's attention unmistakably now.

"What is it?" she asked quickly. "You haven't had bad news?"

An odd smile crossed his face.

"On the contrary." He hesitated a moment, then continued: "I had a longish talk with Dr. McPherson yesterday, and the upshot of it is that I may be required to hand in my checks any day now. I wanted you to know," he added simply.

It was characteristic of the understanding between these two that Patrick made no effort to "break the news," or soften it in any way. He had always been prepared to face facts himself, and he had trained Sara in the same stern creed.

So that now, when he quietly stated in plain language the thing which she had been inwardly dreading for some weeks--for, though silent on the matter, she had not failed to observe his appearance of increasing frailty--she took it like a thorough-bred. Her eyes dilated a little, but her voice was quite steady as she said:

"You mean----"

"I mean that before very long I shall put off this vile body." He glanced down whimsically at his useless legs, cloaked beneath the inevitable rug. "After all," he continued, "life--and death--are both fearfully interesting if one only goes to meet them instead of running away from them. Then they become bogies."

"And what shall I do . . . without you?" she said very low.

"Aye." He nodded. "It's worse for those who are left behind. I've been one of them, and I know. I remember--" He broke off short, his blue eyes dreaming. Presently he gave his shoulders the characteristic little shake which presaged the dismissal of some recalcitrant secret thought, and went on in quick, practical tones.

"I don't want to go out leaving a lot of loose ends behind me--a tangle for you to unravel. So, since the fiat has gone forth--McPherson's a sound man and knows his job--let's face it together, little old pal. It will mean your leaving Barrow, you know," he added tentatively.

Sara nodded, her face rather white.

"Yes, I know. I shan't care--then."

"Oh yes, you will"--with shrewd wisdom. "It will be an extra drop in the bucket, you'll find, when the time comes. Unfortunately, however, there's no getting round the entail, and when I go, my cousin, Major Durward, will reign in my stead."

"Why does the Court go to a Durward?" asked Sara listlessly. "Aren't there any Lovells to inherit?"

"He is a Lovell. His father and mine were brothers, but his godfather, old Timothy Durward left him his property on condition that he adopted the name. Geoffrey

Durward has a son called Timothy--after the old man."

"The Durwards have never been here since I came to live with you," observed Sara thoughtfully. "Don't you care for him--your cousin, I mean?"

"Geoffrey? Yes, he's a charming fellow, and he's been a rattling good soldier-- got his D.S.O. in the South African campaign. But he and his wife--she was a Miss Eden--were stationed in India so many years, I rather lost touch with them. They came home when the Durward property fell in to them--about seven or eight years ago. She, I think"--reminiscently--"was one of the most beautiful women I've ever seen."

The shadow in Sara's eyes lifted for a moment.

"Is that the reason you've always remained a bachelor?" she asked, twinkling.

"God bless my soul, no! I never wanted to marry Elisabeth Eden--though there were plenty of men who did." He regarded Sara with an odd smile. "Some day, you'll know--why I never wanted to marry Elisabeth."

"Tell me now."

He shook his head.

"No. You'll know soon enough--soon enough."

He was silent, fallen a-dreaming once again; and again he seemed to pull himself up short, forcing himself back to the consideration of the practical needs of the moment.

"As I was saying, Sara, sooner or later you'll have to turn out of the old Court. It's entailed, and the income with it. But I've a clear four hundred a year, altogether apart from the Barrow moneys, and that, at my death, will be yours."

"I don't want to hear about it!" burst out Sara passionately. "It's hateful even talking of such things."

Patrick smiled, amused and a little touched by youth's lack of worldly wisdom.

"Don't be a fool, my dear. I shan't die a day sooner for having made my will-- and I shall die a deal more comfortably, knowing that you are provided for. I prom- ised your mother that, as far as lay in my power, I would shield you from wrecking your life as she wrecked hers. And money--a secure little income of her own--is a very good sort of shield for a women. Four hundred's not enough to satisfy a merce- nary individual, but it's enough to enable a woman to marry for love--and not for a home!" He spoke with a kind of repressed bitterness, as though memory had stirred into fresh flame the embers of some burnt-out passion of regret, and Sara looked at him with suddenly aroused interest.

But apparently Patrick did not sense the question that troubled on her lips, or, if he did, had no mind to answer it, for he went on in lighter tones:

"There, that's enough about business for the present. I only wanted you to know that, whatever happens, you will be all right as far as bread-and-cheese are concerned."

"I believe you think that's all I should care about!" exclaimed Sara stormily.

Patrick smiled. He had not been a citizen of the world for over sixty years without acquiring the grim knowledge that neither intense happiness nor deep grief suffice to deaden for very long the pinpricks of material discomfort. But the worldly-wise old man possessed a broad tolerance for the frailties of human nature, and his smile held nothing of contempt, but only a whimsical humour touched with kindly understanding.

"I know you better than that, my dear," he answered quietly. "But I often think of what I once heard an old working-woman, down in the village, say. She had just lost her husband, and the rector's wife was handing out the usual platitudes, and holding forth on the example of Christian fortitude exhibited by a very wealthy lady in the neighbourhood, who had also been recently widowed. 'That's all very well, ma'am,' said my old woman drily, 'but fat sorrow's a deal easier to bear than lean sorrow.' And though it may sound unromantic, it's the raw truth--only very few people are sincere enough to acknowledge it."

In the weeks that followed, Patrick seemed to recover a large measure of his accustomed vigour. He was extraordinarily alert and cheerful--so *alive* that Sara began to hope Dr. McPherson had been mistaken in his opinion, and that there might yet remain many more good years of the happy comradeship that existed between herself and her guardian.

Such buoyancy appeared incompatible with the imminence of death, and one day, driven by the very human instinct to hear her optimism endorsed, she scoffed a little, tentatively, at the doctor's verdict.

Patrick shook his head.

"No, my dear, he's right," he said decisively. "But I'm not going to whine about it. Taken all round, I've found life a very good sort of thing--although"--reflectively--"I've missed the best it has to offer a man. And probably I'll find death a very good sort of thing, too, when it comes."

And so Patrick Lovell went forward, his spirit erect, to meet death with the same cheerful, half-humorous courage he had opposed to the emergencies of life.

It was a few days after this, on Christmas Eve, that Sara, coming into his special den with a gay little joke on her lips and a great bunch of mistletoe in her arms, was arrested by the sudden, chill quiet of the little room.

The familiar wheeled chair was drawn up to the window, and she could see the back of Patrick's head with its thick crop of grizzled hair, but he did not turn or speak at the sound of her entrance.

"Uncle, didn't you hear me? Are you asleep? . . . **Uncle!**" Her voice shrilled on to a sharp staccato note, then cracked and broke suddenly.

There came no movement from the chair. The silence remained unbroken save for the ticking of a clock and the loud beating of her own heart. The two seemed to merge into one gigantic pulse . . . deafening . . . overwhelming . . . like the surge of some immense, implacable sea.

She swayed a little, clutching at the door for support. Then the throbbing ceased, and she was only conscious of a solitude so intense that it seemed to press about her like a tangible thing.

Swiftly, on feet of terror, she crossed the room and stood looking down at the motionless figure of her uncle. His face was turned towards the sun, and wore an expression of complete happiness and content, as though he had just found something for which he had been searching. He had looked like that a thousand times, when, seeking for her, he had come upon her, at last, hidden in some shady nook in the garden or swinging in her hammock. She could almost hear the familiar "Oh, there you are, little pal!" with which he would joyously acclaim her discovery.

She lifted the hand that was resting quietly on his knee. It lay in hers, flaccid and inert, its dreadful passivity stinging her into realization of the truth. Patrick was dead. And, judging from his expression, he had found death "a very good sort of thing," just as he had expected.

For a little while Sara remained standing quietly beside the still figure in the chair. They would never be alone together any more--not quite like this, Patrick sitting in his accustomed place, wearing his beloved old tweeds, with an immaculate tie and with his single eyeglass--about which she had so often chaffed him--dangling across his chest on its black ribbon.

Her mouth quivered. "Stand up to it!" . . . The voice--Patrick's voice--seemed to sound in her ear . . . "Stand up to it, little old pal!"

She bit back the sob that climbed to her throat, and stood silently facing the enemy, as it were.

This was the end, then, of one chapter of her existence--the chapter of sheltered, happy life at Barrow, and in these quiet moments, alone for the last time with Patrick Lovell, Sara tried to gather strength and courage from her memories of his cheery optimism to face gamely whatever might befall her in the big world into which she must so soon adventure.

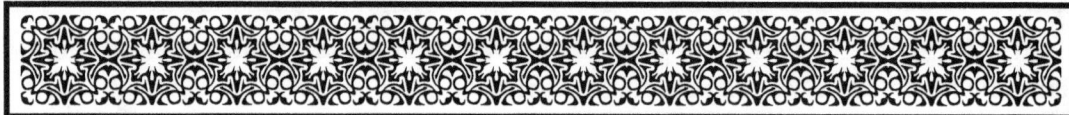

CHAPTER III
A SHEAF OF MEMORIES

It was over. The master of Barrow had been carried shoulder-high to the great vault where countless Lovells slept their last sleep, the blinds had been drawn up, letting in the wintry sunlight once again, and the mourners had gone their ways. Only the new owner of the Court still lingered, and even he would be leaving very soon now.

Sara, her slim, boyish build, with its long line of slender hip, accentuated by the clinging black of her gown, moved listlessly across the hall to where Major Durward was standing smoking by the big open fire, waiting for the car which was to take him to the station.

He made as though to throw his cigarette away at her approach, but she gestured a hasty negative.

"No, don't," she said. "I like it. It seems to make things a little more natural. Uncle Pat"--with a wan smile--"was always smoking."

Her sombre eyes were shadowed and sad, and there was a pinched, drawn look about her nostrils. Major Durward regarded her with a concerned expression on his kindly face.

"You will miss him badly," he said.

"Yes, I shall miss him,"--simply. She returned his glance frankly. "You are very like him, you know," she added suddenly.

It was true. The big, soldierly man beside her, with his jolly blue eyes, grey hair, and short-clipped military moustache, bore a striking resemblance to the Patrick Lovell of ten years ago, before ill-health had laid its finger upon him, and during the difficult days that succeeded her uncle's death Sara had unconsciously found a strange kind of comfort in the likeness. She had dreaded inexpressibly the advent of the future owner of Barrow, but, when he had arrived, his resemblance to his dead cousin, and a certain similarity of gesture and of voice, common enough in families, had at once established a sense of kinship, which had deepened with her recognition of Durward's genuine kind-heartedness and solicitude for her comfort.

He had immediately assumed control of affairs, taking all the inevitable detail of arrangement off her shoulders, yet deferring to her as though she were still just as much mistress of the Court as she had been before her uncle's death. In every way he had tried to ease and smooth matters for her, and she felt proportionately grateful to him.

"Then, if you think I'm like him," said Durward gently, "will you let me try to take his place a little? I mean," he explained hastily, fearing she might misunderstand him, "that you will miss his guardianship and care of you, as well as the good pal you found in him. Will you let me try to fill in the gaps, if--if you should want advice, or service--anything over which a male man can be a bit useful? Oh----" breaking off with a short, embarrassed laugh--"it is so difficult to explain what I do mean!"

"I think I know," said Sara, smiling faintly. "You mean that now that Uncle Pat has gone, you don't want me to feel quite adrift in the world."

The big man, hampered by his masculine shyness of a difficult situation, smiled back at her, relieved.

"Yes, that's it, that's it!" he agreed eagerly. "I want you to regard me as a--a sort of sheet-anchor upon which you can pull in a storm."

"Thank you," said Sara. "I will. But I hope there won't be storms of such magnitude that I shall need to pull very hard."

Durward smoked furiously for a moment. Then he burst forth--

"You can't imagine what a brute I feel for turning you out of the Court. I wish it need not be. But the Lovells have always lived at the old place, and my wife--"

"Naturally." She interrupted him gently. "Naturally, she wishes to live here. I owe you no grudge for that," smiling. "When--how soon do you think of coming? I will make my arrangements accordingly."

"We should like to come as soon as possible, really," he admitted reluctantly. "I have the chance of leasing Durward Park, if the tenant can have what practically amounts to immediate possession. And of course, in the circumstances, I should be glad to get the Durward property off my hands."

"Of course you would." Sara nodded understandingly. "If you could let me have a few days in which to find some rooms--"

"No, no," he broke in eagerly. "I want you still to regard Barrow as your head-quarters--to stay on here with us until you have fixed some permanent arrangement that suits you."

She was touched by the kindly suggestion; nevertheless, she shook her head with decision.

"It is more than kind of you to think of such a thing," she said gratefully. "But it is quite out of the question. Why, I am not even a cousin several times removed! I have no claim at all. Mrs. Durward--"

"Will be delighted. She asked me to be sure and tell you so. Please, Miss Tennant, don't refuse me. Don't"--persuasively--"oblige us to feel more brutal interlopers than we need."

Still she hesitated.

"If I were sure--" she began doubtfully.

"You may be--absolutely sure. There!"--with a sigh of relief--"that's settled. But, as I can see you're the kind of person whose conscientious scruples will begin to worry you the moment I'm gone"--he smiled--"my wife will write to you. Promise not to run away in the meantime?"

"I promise," said Sara. She held out her hand. "And--thank you." Her eyes, suddenly misty, supplemented the baldness of the words.

He took the outstretched hand in a close, friendly grip.

"Good. That's the car, I think," as the even purring of a motor sounded from outside. "I must be off. But it's only *au revoir*, remember."

She walked with him to the door, and stood watching until the car was lost in sight round a bend of the drive. Then, as she turned back into the hall, the emptiness of the house seemed to close down about her all at once, like a pall.

Amid the manifold duties and emergencies of the last few days she had hardly had time to realize the immensity of her loss. Practical matters had forcibly obtruded themselves upon her consideration--the necessity of providing accommodation for the various relatives who had attended the funeral, the frequent consultations that Major Durward, to all intents and purposes a stranger to the ways of Barrow, had been obliged to hold with her, the reading of the will--all these had combined to keep her in a state of mental and physical alertness which had mercifully precluded retrospective thought.

But now the necessity for *doing* anything was past; there were no longer any claims upon her time, nothing to distract her, and she had leisure to visualize the full significance of Patrick's death and all that it entailed.

Rather languidly she mounted the stairs to her own room, and drawing up a low chair to the fire, sat staring absently into its glowing heart.

Virtually, she was alone in the world. Even Major Durward, who had been so infinitely kind, was not bound to her by any ties other than those forged of his own friendly feelings. True, he had been Patrick's cousin. But Patrick, although he had made up Sara's whole world, had been entirely unrelated to her.

Her heart throbbed with a sudden rush of intense gratitude towards the man who had so amply fulfilled his trust as guardian, and she glanced up wistfully at the big photograph of him which stood upon the chimney-piece.

Propped against the photo-frame was a square white envelope on which was written: *To be given to my ward, Sara Tennant, after my death*. The family solicitor had handed it to her the previous day, after the reading of the will, but the demands upon her time and attention had been so many, owing to the number of relatives who temporarily filled the house, that she had laid it on one side for perusal when she should be alone once more.

The sight of the familiar handwriting brought a swift mist of tears to her eyes, and she hesitated a little before opening the sealed envelope.

It was strange to realize that here was some message for her from Patrick himself, but that no matter what the envelope might contain, she would be able to give back no answer, make no reply. The knowledge seemed to set him very far away from her, and for a few moments she sobbed quietly, feeling utterly solitary and alone.

Presently she brushed the tears from her eyes and slit open the flap of the envelope. Inside was a half-sheet of notepaper wrapped about a small old-fashioned key, and on the outer fold was written: "*The key of the Chippendale bureau*." That was all.

For an instant Sara was puzzled. Then she remembered that amongst Patrick's personal bequests to her had been that of the small mahogany bureau which stood near the window of his bedroom. It had not occurred to her at the time that its contents might have any interest for her; in fact, she had supposed it to be empty. But now she realized that there was evidently something within it which Patrick must have valued, seeing he had guarded the key so carefully and directed its delivery to her through the reliable hands of his solicitor.

Rather glad of anything that might help to occupy her thoughts, she decided to investigate the bureau at once, and accordingly made her way to Patrick's bedroom.

On the threshold she paused, her heart contracting painfully as the spick and span aspect of the room, its ordered absence of any trace of occupation, reminded her that its one-time owner would never again have any further need of it.

Everything in the house seemed to present her grief to her anew, from some fresh angle, forcing comparison of what had been with what was--the wheeled chair, standing vacant in one of the lobbies, the tobacco jar perched upon the chimney-piece, the pot of heliotrope--Patrick's favourite blossom--scenting the library with its fragrance.

And now his room--empty, swept, and garnished like any one of the score or so of spare bedrooms in the house!

With an effort, Sara forced herself to enter it. Crossing to the window, she pulled a chair up to the Chippendale bureau and unlocked it. Then she drew out the sliding desk supports and laid back the flap of polished mahogany that served as a writing-table. She was conscious of a fleeting sense of admiration for the fine-grained wood and for the smooth "feel" of the old brass handles, worn by long usage, then her whole attention was riveted by the three things which were all the contents of the desk--a packet of letters, stained and yellowing with age and tied together with a broad, black ribbon, a jeweller's velvet case stamped with faded gilt lettering, and an envelope addressed to herself in Patrick's handwriting.

Very gently, with that tender reverence we accord to the sad little possessions of our dead, Sara gathered them up and carried them to her own sitting-room. She felt she could not stay to examine them in that strangely empty, lifeless room that had been Patrick's; the terrible, chill silence of it seemed to beat against the very heart of her.

Laying aside the jeweller's case and the package of letters, she opened the envelope which bore her name and drew out a folded sheet of paper, covered with Patrick's small, characteristic writing. Impulsively she brushed it with her lips, then, leaning back in her chair, began to read, her expression growing curiously intent as she absorbed the contents of the letter. Once she smiled, and more than once a sudden rush of unbidden tears blurred the closely written lines in front of her.

"When you receive this, little pal Sara"--ran the letter--"I shall have done with this world. Except that it means leaving you, my dear, I shall be glad to go, for I'm a very tired man. So, when it comes, you must try not to grudge me my 'long leave.' But there are several things you ought to know, and which I want you to know, yet I have never been able to bring myself to speak of them to you. To tell you about them meant digging into the past--and very often there is a hot coal lingering in the heart of a dead fire that is apt to burn the fingers of whoever rakes out the ashes. Frankly, then, I funked it. But now the time has come when I can't put it off any longer.

"Little old pal, have you ever wondered why I loved you so much--why you stood so close to my heart? I used to tease you and say it was because we were no relation to each other, didn't I? If you had been really my niece, proper respect (on your part, of course, for your aged uncle!) and the barrier of a generation would have set us the usual miles apart. But there was never anything of that with us, was there? I bullied you, I know, when you needed it, but we were always comrades. And to me, you were something more than a comrade, something almost sacred and always adorable--the child of the woman I loved.

"For we should have been married, Sara, your mother and I, had I not been a poor man. We were engaged, but at that time, I was only a younger son, with a younger son's meager portion, and the prospect of my falling heir to Barrow seemed of all things the most improbable. And Pauline Malincourt, your mother, had been taught to abhor the idea of living on small means--trained to regard her beauty and breeding as marketable assets, to go to the highest bidder. For, although her parents came of fine old stock--there's no better blood in England than the Malincourt strain, my dear--they were deadly hard-up. So hard-up, that when they died--as the result of a carriage accident which occurred a week after Pauline's marriage--they left nothing behind them but debts which your father liquidated.

"Of your father, Caleb Tennant, the millionaire, I will not write, seeing that, after all, you are his child. It is enough to say that he was a hard man, and that he and your mother led a very unhappy life together, so unhappy that at last she left him, choosing rather to live in utter poverty than remain with him. He never forgave her for leaving him, and when he died, he willed every penny he possessed to some scoundrelly cousin of his--who is presumably enjoying the inheritance which should have been yours.

"That is your family history, my dear, and it is right that you should know it--and know what you have to fight against. To be a Malincourt is at once to have a curse and a blessing hung round your neck. The Malincourts were originally of French extraction--descendants of the **haute noblesse** of old France--cursed with the devil's own pride and passionate self-will, and blessed with looks and brains and charm above the average. They never bend; they break sooner. And I think you've got the lot, Sara--the full inheritance.

"Your mother was a true Malincourt. She could not bend, and when things went awry, she broke.

"You must never think hardly of her, for she had been brought up in that atmosphere of almost desperate pride which is too frequently the curse of the poverty-stricken aristocrat. She made a ghastly mistake, and paid for it afterwards every day of her life. And she was urged into it by her father, who declined to recognize me in any way, and by her mother, who made her life at home a simple hell--as a clever society woman can make of any young girl's life if she chooses.

"Just before she died, she sent for me and gave you into my care, begging me to shield you from spoiling your life as she had spoiled hers.

"I've done what I could. You are at least independent. No one can drive you with the spur of poverty into selling yourself, as she was driven. But there are a hundred other rocks in life against which you may wreck your happiness, and remember, in the long run, you sink or swim by your own force of character.

"And when love comes to you, **as it will come**,--for no woman with your eyes and your mouth ever yet lived a loveless life!--never forget that it is the biggest thing in the world, the one altogether good and perfect gift. Don't let any twopenny-halfpenny considerations of worldly advantage influence you, nor the tittle-tattle of other folks, and even if it seems that something insurmountable lies between you and the fulfillment of love, go over it, or round it, or through it! If it's a real love, your faith must be big enough to remove the mountains in the way--or to go over them.

"The package of letters you will find in the bureau were those your mother wrote to me during the few short weeks we belonged to each other. I'm a senti-mental old fool, and I've never been able to bring myself to burn them. Will you do this for me?

"In the little velvet case you will find her miniature, which I give to you. It is very like her--and like you, too, for you resemble her wonderfully in appearance. Often, to look at you has made my heart ache; sometimes it almost seemed as if the years had rolled back and Pauline herself stood before me.

"And now that the order for release is on its way to me, it is rather wonderful to reflect that in a few weeks--a few days, perhaps--I shall be seeing her again. . . .

"Good-bye, little pal of mine. We've had some good times together, haven't we?

"Your devoted, PATRICK."

Sara sat very still, the letter clasped in her hand. She had always secretly be-lieved that some long-dead romance lay behind Patrick's bachelorhood, but she had never suspected that her own mother had been the woman he had loved.

The knowledge illumined all the past with a fresh light, investing it with a tender, reminiscent sentiment. It was easy now to understand the almost idyllic atmosphere Patrick had infused into their life together. Sara recognized it as the outcome of a love and fidelity as beautiful and devoted as it is rare. Patrick's love for her mother had partaken of the enduring qualities of the great passions of history. Paolo and Francesca, Abelard and Heloise--even they could have known no deeper, no more lasting love than that of Patrick Lovell for Pauline.

The love-letters of the dead woman lay on Sara's lap, still tied together with the black ribbon which Patrick's fingers must have knotted round them. There were only six of them--half-a-dozen memories of a love that had come hopelessly to grief--tangible memories which her lover had never had the heart to destroy.

Sara handled them caressingly, these few, pathetic records of a bygone passion, and at length, with hands that shook a little, she removed the ribbon that bound them together. Where it had lain, preserving the strip of paper beneath it from contact with the dust, bands of white traversed the faint discoloration which time had worked upon the outermost envelopes--mutely witnessing to the long years that had passed away since the letters had been penned in the first rapturous glow of hot young love.

Slowly, with a rather wistful sense of regret that it must needs be done, Sara dropped them one by one, unread, into the fire, and watched them flare up with a sudden spurt of flame, then curl and shrivel into dead, grey ash--those last links with the romance of his youth which Patrick had treasured so long and faithfully.

She wondered what manner of woman her mother could have been to inspire so great a love that even her own unfaith had failed to sour it. Her childish recollection, blurred by the passage of years, was of a white-faced, rather haggard-looking woman with deep-set, haunted eyes and a bitter mouth, but whose rare smile, when it came, was so enchanting that it wiped out, for the moment, all remembrance of the harsh lines which hardened her face when in repose.

With eager hands the girl picked up the little velvet case that held the miniature, and snapped open the lid. The painting within, rimmed in old paste, was of a girl in her early twenties. The face was oval, with a small, pointed chin and a vivid red mouth, curling up at the corners. There was little colour in the cheeks, and the black hair and extraordinarily dark eyes served to enhance the creamy pallor of the skin. It was not altogether an English face; the cheek-bones were too high, and there was a definiteness of colouring, a decisive sharpness of outline in the piquant features, not often found in a purely English type.

Seen thus, the face looked strangely familiar to Sara, and yet no memory of hers could recall her mother as she must have been at the time this portrait was painted.

The miniature still in her hand, she moved hesitatingly to a mirror, so placed that the light from the window fell full upon her as she faced it. In a moment the odd sense of familiarity was explained. There, looking back at her from the mirror, was the same sharply angled face, the same warm ivory pallor of complexion, accentuated by raven hair and black, sombre eyes. What was it Patrick had written? *"No woman with your eyes and your mouth ever yet lived a loveless life."*

With a curious deliberation, Sara examined the features in question. The eyes were long, and the lids, opaquely white and fringed with jet-black lashes, slanted downwards a little at the outer corners, bestowing a curiously intense expression, such as one sometimes sees in the eyes of an actor, and the mouth was the same vividly scarlet mouth of the face in the miniature, at once passionate and sensitive.

The French strain in the Malincourt family had reproduced itself indubitably, both in the appearance of Pauline and of Pauline's daughter. Would the mother's tragedy, fruit of her singular charm and of a pride which had accorded love but a secondary place in her scheme of life, also be re-enacted in the case of the daughter? It seemed almost as though Patrick must have had pre-vision of some like fiery ordeal though which his "little old pal" might have to pass, so urgent had been the warning he had uttered.

Sara shivered, as if she, too, felt a prescience of coming disaster. It was as though a shadow had fallen across her path, a shadow of which the substance lay hidden, shrouded in the mists which veil the future.

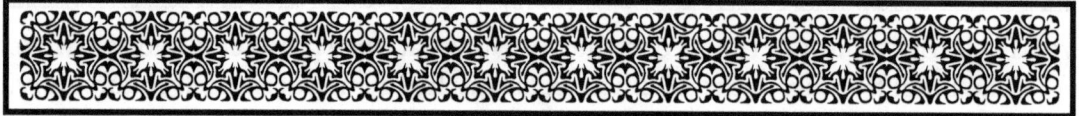

CHAPTER IV
ELISABETH--AND HER SON

The entrance to Barrow Court was somewhat forbidding. A flight of shallow granite steps, flanked by balustrades of the same austere substance, terminating in huge, rough-hewn pillars, led up to an enormous door of ancient oak, studded with nails--destined, it would seem, to resist the onslaught of an armed multitude. The sternness of its aspect, when the great door was closed, seemed to add an increased warmth to the suggestion of welcome it conveyed when, as now, it was swung hospitably open, emitting a ruddy glow of firelight from the hall beyond.

Sara was standing at the top of the granite steps, waiting to greet the Durwards, whose approach was already heralded by the humming of a motor far down the avenue.

A faint regret disquieted her. This was the last--the very last--time she would stand at the head of those stairs in the capacity of a hostess welcoming her guests; and even now her position there was merely an honorary one! In a few minutes, when Mrs. Durward should step across the threshold, it was she who would be transformed into the hostess, while Sara would have to take her place as a simple guest in the house which for twelve years had been her home.

Thrusting the thought determinedly aside, she watched the big limousine swing smoothly round the curve of the drive and pull up in front of the house, and there was no trace of reluctance in the smile of greeting which she summoned up for Major Durward's benefit as he alighted and came towards her with outstretched hand.

"But where are the others?" asked Sara, seeing that the chauffeur immediately headed the car for the garage.

"They're coming along on foot," explained Durward. "Elisabeth declared they should see nothing of the place cooped up in the car, so they got out at the lodge and are walking across the park."

Sara preceded him into the hall, and they stood chatting together by the tea-table until the sound of voices announced the arrival of the rest of the party.

"Here they are!" exclaimed Durward, hurrying forward to meet them, while Sara followed a trifle hesitatingly, conscious of a sudden accession of shyness.

Notwithstanding the charming letter she had received from Mrs. Durward, begging her to remain at Barrow Court exactly as long as it suited her, now that the moment had come which would actually install the new mistress of the Court, she began to feel as though her continued presence there might be regarded rather in the light of an intrusion.

Mrs. Durward's letter might very well have been dictated only by a certain superficial politeness, or, even, solely at the instance of her husband, and it was conceivable that the writer would be none too pleased that her invitation had been so literally interpreted.

In the course of a few seconds of time Sara contrived to work herself up into a condition bordering upon panic. And then a very low contralto voice, indescribably sweet, and with an audacious ripple of laughter running through it, swept all her scruples into the rubbish heap. There was no doubting the sincerity of the speaker.

"It was so nice of you not to run away, Miss Tennant." As she spoke, Mrs. Durward shook hands cordially. "Poor Geoffrey couldn't help being the heir, you know, and if you'd refused to stay, he'd have felt just like the villain in a cinema film. You've saved us from becoming the crawling, self-reproachful wretches." Then she turned and beckoned to her son. "This is Tim," she said simply, but the quality of her voice was very much as though she had announced: "This is the sun, and moon, and stars."

As mother and son stood side by side, Sara's first impression was that she had never seen two more beautiful people. They were both tall, and a kind of radiance seemed to envelope them--a glory imparted by the sheer force of perfect symmetry and health--and, in the case of the former of the two, there was an added charm in a certain little air of stateliness and distinction which characterized her movements.

Patrick's reminiscent comment on Elisabeth Durward recalled itself to Sara's mind: "I think she was one of the most beautiful women I have ever seen," and she recognized that almost any one might have truthfully subscribed to the same opinion.

Mrs. Durward must have been at least forty years of age--arguing from the presence of the six foot of young manhood whom she called son--but her appearance was still that of a woman who had not long passed her thirtieth milestone. The supple lines of her figure held the merest suggestion of maturity in their gracious curves, and the rich chestnut hair, swathed round her small, fine head, gleamed with the sheen which only youth or immense vitality bestows. Her skin was of that almost dazzling purity which is so often found in conjunction with reddish hair, and the defect of over-light brows and lashes, which not infrequently mars the type, was conspicuously absent. Her eyes were arresting. They were of a deep, hyacinth blue, very luminous and soft, and quite beautiful. But they held a curiously veiled expression--a something guarded and inscrutable--as though they hid some secret inner knowledge sentinelled from the world at large.

Sara, meeting their still, enigmatic gaze, was subtly conscious of an odd sense of repulsion, almost amounting to dread, and then Elisabeth, making some trivial observation as she moved nearer to the fire, smiled across at her, and, in the extraordinary charm of her smile, the momentary sensation of fear was forgotten.

Nevertheless, it was with a feeling of relief that Sara encountered the gay, frank glance of the son.

Tim Durward, though dowered to the full with his mother's beauty, had yet been effectually preserved from the misfortune of being an effeminate repetition of her. In him, Elisabeth's glowing auburn colouring had sobered to a steady brown--evidenced in the crisp, curly hair and sun-tanned skin; and the misty hyacinth-blue of her eyes had hardened in the eyes of her son into the clear, bright azure of the sea, whist the beautiful contours of her face, repeated in his, had strengthened into a fine young virility.

"I can't cure mother of introducing me as if I were the Lord Mayor," he murmured plaintively to Sara as they sat down to tea. "I suppose it's the penalty of being an only son."

"Nothing of the sort," asserted Elisabeth composedly. "Naturally I'm pleased with you--you're so absurdly like me. I always look upon you in the light of a perpetual compliment, because you've elected to grow up like me instead of like Geoffrey"--nodding towards her husband. "After all, you had us both to choose from."

Tim shouted with delight.

"Listen to her, Miss Tennant! And for years I've been mistaking mere vulgar female vanity for maternal solicitude."

"Anyway, you're a very poor compliment," threw in Major Durward, with an expressive glance at his wife's beautiful face. It was obvious that he worshipped her, and she smiled across at him, blushing adorably, just like a girl of sixteen.

Tim turned to Sara with a grimace.

"It's a great trial, Miss Tennant, to be blessed with two parents--"

"It's quite usual," interpolated Geoffrey mildly.

"Two parents," continued Tim, firmly ignoring him, "who are hopelessly, besottedly in love with each other. Instead of being--as I ought to be--the apple of their eye--of both their eyes--I'm merely the shadowy third."

Sara surveyed his goodly proportions consideringly.

"No one would have suspected it," she assured him; and Tim grinned appreciatively.

"If you stay with us long," he replied, "as I hope"--impressively--"you will, you'll soon perceive how utterly I am neglected. Perhaps"--his face brightening--"you may be moved to take pity on my solitude--quite frequently."

"Tim, stop being an idiot," interposed his mother placidly, holding out her cup, "and ask Miss Tennant to give me another lump of sugar."

The advent of the Durwards, breaking in upon her enforced solitude, helped very considerably to arouse Sara from the natural depression into which she had fallen after Patrick's death. With their absurdly large share of good looks, their charmingly obvious attachment to each other, and their enthusiastic, unconventional hospitality towards such an utter stranger as herself, devoid of any real claim upon them, she found the trio unexpectedly interesting and delightful. They had hailed her as a friend, and her frank, warm-hearted nature responded instantly, speedily according each of them a special niche in her regard. She felt as though Providence had suddenly endowed her with a whole family--"all complete and ready for use," as Tim cheerfully observed--and the reaction from the oppressive consciousness of being entirely alone in the world acted like a tonic.

The first brief sentiment of aversion which she had experienced towards Elisabeth melted like snow in sunshine under the daily charm of her companionship; and though the hyacinth eyes held always in their depths that strange suggestion of mystery, Sara grew to believe it must be merely some curious effect incidental to the colour and shape of the eyes themselves, rather than an indication of the soul that looked out of them.

There was something perennially captivating about Elisabeth. An atmosphere of romance enveloped her, engendering continuous interest and surmise, and Sara found it wholly impossible to view her from an ordinary prosaic standpoint. Occasionally she would recall the fact that Mrs. Durward was in reality a woman of over forty, mother of a grown-up son who, according to all the usages of custom, should be settling down into the drab and placid backwater of middle age, but she realized that the description went ludicrously wide of the mark.

There was nothing in the least drab about Elisabeth, nor would there ever be. She was full of colour and brilliance, reminding one of a great glowing-hearted rose in its prime.

Part of her charm, undoubtedly, lay in her attitude towards husband and son. She was still as romantically in love with Major Durward as any girl in her teens, and she adored Tim quite openly.

Inevitably, perhaps, there was a touch of the spoilt woman about her, since both men combined to indulge her in every whim. Nevertheless, there was nothing either small or petty in her willfulness. It was rather the superb, stately arrogance of a queen, and she was kindness itself to Sara.

But the largest share of credit in restoring the latter to a more normal and less highly strung condition was due to Tim, who gravitated towards her with the facility common to natural man when he finds himself for any length of time under the same roof with an attractive young person of the opposite sex. He had an engaging habit of appearing at the door of Sara's sitting-room with an ingratiating: "I say, may I come in for a yarn?" And, upon receiving permission, he would establish himself on the hearth-rug at her feet and proceed to prattle to her about his own affairs, much as a brother might have done to a favourite sister, and with an equal assurance that his confidences would be met with sympathetic interest.

"What are you going to do with yourself, Tim?" asked Sara one day, as he sprawled in blissful indolence on the great bearskin in front of her fire, pulling happily at a beloved old pipe.

"Do with myself?" he repeated. "What do you mean? I'm doing very comfortably just at present"--glancing round him appreciatively.

"I mean--what are you going to be? Aren't you going to enter any profession?"

Tim sat up suddenly, removing his pipe from his mouth.

"No," he said shortly.

"But why not? You can't slack about here for ever, doing nothing. I should have thought you would have gone into the Army, like your father."

His blue eyes hardened.

"That's what I wanted to do," he said gruffly. "But the mother wouldn't hear of it."

Sara could sense the pain in his suddenly roughened tones.

"But why? You'd make a splendid soldier, Tim"--eyeing his long length affectionately.

"I should have loved it," he said wistfully. "I wanted it more than anything. But mother worried so frightfully whenever I suggested the idea that I had to give it up. I'm to learn to be a landowner and squire and all that sort of tosh instead."

"But that could come later."

Tim shrugged his shoulders.

"Of course it could. But mother refused point-blank to let me go to Sandhurst. So now, unless a war crops up--and it doesn't look as though there's much chance of that!--I'm out of the running. But if it ever does, Sara"--he laid his hand eagerly on her knee--"I swear I'll be one of the first to volunteer. I was a fool to give in to the mother over the matter, only she was simply making herself ill about it, and, of course, I couldn't stand that."

Sara wondered why Mrs. Durward should have interfered to prevent her son from following what was obviously his natural bent. It would have seemed almost inevitable that, as a soldier's son, he should enter one or other of the Services, and instead, here he was, stranded in a little country backwater, simply eating his heart out. Mentally she determined to broach the subject to Elisabeth as soon as an opportunity presented itself; but for the moment she skillfully drew the conversation away from what was evidently a sore subject, and suggested that Tim should accompany her into Fallowdene, where she had an errand at the post office. He assented eagerly, with a shake of his broad shoulders as though to rid himself of the disagreeable burden of his thoughts.

From the window of his wife's sitting-room Major Durward watched the two as they started on their way to the village, evidently on the best of terms with one another, a placid smile spreading beneficently over his face as they vanished round the corner of the shrubbery.

"Anything in it, do you think?" he asked, seeing that Elisabeth's gaze had pursued the same course.

"It's impossible to say," she answered quietly. "Tim imagines himself to be falling in love, I don't doubt; but at twenty-two a boy imagines himself in love with half the girls he meets."

"I didn't," declared Geoffrey promptly. "I fell in love with you at the mature age of nineteen--and I never fell out again."

Elisabeth flashed him a charming smile.

"Perhaps Tim may follow in your footsteps, then," she suggested serenely.

"Well, would you be pleased?" persisted her husband, jerking his head explanatorily in the direction in which Sara and Tim had disappeared.

"I shall always be pleased with the woman who makes Tim happy," she answered simply.

Durward was silent a moment; then he returned to the attack.

"She's a very pretty young woman, don't you think?"

"Sara? No, I shouldn't call her exactly pretty. Her face is too thin, and strong, and eager. But she is a very uncommon type--like a black and white etching, and immensely attractive."

It was several days before Sara was able to introduce the topic of Tim's profession, but she contrived it one afternoon when she and Elisabeth were sitting together awaiting the return of the two men for tea.

"It will be profession enough for Tim to look after the property," Elisabeth made answer. "He can act as agent for his father to some extent, and relieve him of a great deal of necessary business that has to be transacted."

She spoke with a certain finality which made it difficult to pursue the subject, but Sara, remembering Tim's suddenly hard young eyes, persisted.

"It's a pity he cannot go into the Army--he's so keen on it," she suggested tentatively.

A curious change came over Elisabeth's face. It seemed to Sara as though a veil had descended, from behind which the inscrutable eyes were watching her warily. But the response was given lightly enough.

"Oh, one of the family in the Service is enough. I should see so little of my Tim if he became a soldier--only an occasional 'leave.'"

"He would make a very good soldier," said Sara. "To my mind, it's the finest profession in the world for any man."

"Do you think so?" Elisabeth spoke coldly. "There are many risks attached to it."

Sara experienced a revulsion of feeling; she had not expected Elisabeth to be of the fearful type of woman. Women of splendid physique and abounding vitality are rarely obsessed by craven apprehensions.

"I don't think the risks would count with Tim," she said warmly. "He has any amount of pluck." And then she stared at Elisabeth in amazement. A sudden haggardness had overspread the elder woman's face, the faint shell-pink that usually flushed her cheeks draining away and leaving them milk-white.

"Yes," she replied in stifled tones. "I don't suppose Tim's a coward. But"--more lightly--"I think I am. I--don't think I care for the Army as a profession. Tim is my only child," she added self-excusingly. "I can't let him run risks--of any kind."

As she spoke, an odd foreboding seized hold of Sara. It was as though the secret dread of ***something***--she could not tell what--which held the mother had communicated itself to her.

She shivered. Then, the impression fading as quickly as it had come, she spoke defiantly, as if trying to reassure herself.

"There aren't many risks in these piping times of peace. Soldiers don't die in battle nowadays; they retire on a pension."

"Die in battle! Did you think I was afraid of that?" There was a sudden fierce contempt in Elisabeth's voice.

Sara looked at her with astonishment.

"Weren't you?" she said hesitatingly.

Elisabeth seemed about to make some passionate rejoinder. Then, all at once, she checked herself, and again Sara was conscious of that curiously secretive expression in her eyes, as though she were on guard.

"There are many things worse than death," she said evasively, and deliberately turned the conversation into other channels.

During the days that followed, Sara became aware of a faintly perceptible difference in her relations with Elisabeth. The latter was still just as charming as ever, but she seemed, in some inexplicable way, to have set a limit to their intimacy--defined a boundary line which she never intended to be overstepped.

It was as though she felt that she had allowed Sara to approach too nearly some inner sanctum which she had hitherto guarded securely from all intrusion, and now hastened to erect a barricade against a repetition of the offence.

More than once, lately, Sara had broached the subject of her impending departure from Barrow, only to have the suggestion incontinently brushed aside by Major Durward, who declared that he declined to discuss any such disagreeable topic. But now, sensitively conscious that she had troubled Elisabeth's peace in some way, she decided to make definite arrangements regarding her immediate future.

She was agreeably surprised, when she propounded her idea, to find Mrs. Durward seemed quite as unwilling to part with her as were both her husband and son. Apparently the alteration in her manner, with its curiously augmented reticence, was no indication of any personal antipathy, and Sara felt proportionately relieved, although somewhat mystified.

"We shall all miss you," averred Elisabeth, and there was absolute sincerity in her tones. "I don't see why you need be in such a hurry to run away from us." And Geoffrey and Tim chorused approval.

Sara beamed upon them all with humid eyes.

"It's dear of you to want me to stay with you," she declared. "But, don't you see, I **must** live my own life--have a roof-tree of my own? I can't just sit down comfortably in the shade of yours."

"Pushful young woman!" chaffed Geoffrey. "Well, I can see your mind is made up. So what are your plans? Let's hear them."

"I thought of taking rooms for a while with some really nice people--gentlefolk who wanted to take a paying guest--"

"Poor but honest, in fact," supplemented Geoffrey.

Sara nodded.

"Yes. You see"--smiling--"you people have spoiled me for living alone, and as I'm really rather a solitary individual, I must find a little niche for myself some-where." She unfolded a letter she was holding. "I thought I should like to go near the sea--to some quite tiny country place at the back of beyond. And I think I've found just the thing. I saw an advertisement for a paying guest--of the female per-suasion--so I replied to it, and I've just had an answer to my letter. It's from a doctor man--a Dr. Selwyn, at Monkshaven--who has an invalid wife and one daughter, and he writes such an original kind of epistle that I'm sure I should like him."

Geoffrey held out his hand for the letter, running his eyes down its contents, while his wife, receiving an assenting nod from Sara in response to her "May I?" looked over his shoulder.

Only Tim appeared to take no interest in the matter, but remained standing rather aloof, staring out of the window, his back to the trio grouped around the hearth.

"'Household . . . myself, wife, one daughter,'" muttered Geoffrey. "Um-um--'quarter of a mile from the sea'--um----'As you will have guessed from the fact of my advertising'"--here he began to read aloud--"'we are not too lavishly blessed with this world's goods. Our house is roomy and comfortable, though abominably furnished. But I can guarantee the climate, and there are plenty of nicer people than ourselves in the neighbourhood. It wouldn't be fitting for me to blow our own particular household trumpet--nor, to tell the truth, is it always calculated to give forth melodious sounds; but if the other considerations I have mentioned commend themselves to you, I suggest that you come down and make trial of us.'"

"Don't you think he sounds just delightful?" queried Sara.

Manlike, Geoffrey shook his head disapprovingly.

"No, I don't," he said decisively. "That's the most unbusinesslike letter I've ever read."

"*I* like it very much," announced Elisabeth with equal decision. "The man writes just as he thinks--perfectly frankly and naturally. I should go and give them a trial as he suggests. Sara, if I were you."

"That's what I feel inclined to do," replied Sara. "I thought it a delicious letter."

Geoffrey shrugged his shoulders resignedly.

"Then, of course, if you two women have made up your minds that the man's a natural saint, I may as well hold my peace. What's the fellow's address?--I'll look him up in the Medical Directory. Richard Selwyn, Sunnyside, Monkshaven--that right?"

He departed to the library in search of Dr. Selywn's credentials, presently returning with a somewhat rueful grin on his face.

"He seems all right--rather a clever man, judging by his degrees and the appointments he has held," he acknowledged grudgingly.

"I'm sure he's all right, asserted Sara firmly.

"Although I don't understand why such a good man at his job should be practicing in a little one-horse place like Monkshaven," retorted Geoffrey maliciously.

"Probably he went there on account of his wife's health," suggested Elisabeth. "He says she is an invalid."

"Oh, well"--Geoffrey yielded unwillingly--"I suppose you'll go, Sara. But if the experiment isn't a success you must come back to us at once. Is that a bargain?"

Sara hesitated.

"Promise," commanded Geoffrey. "Or"--firmly--"I'm hanged if we let you go at all."

"Very well," agreed Sara meekly. "I'll promise."

"I hope the experiment will be an utter failure," observed Tim, later on, when he and Sara were alone together. He spoke with an oddly curt--almost inimical--inflection in his voice.

"Now that's unkind of you, Tim," she protested smilingly. "I thought you were a good enough pal not to want to chortle over me--as I know Geoffrey will--should the thing turn out a frost!"

"Well, I'm not, then," he returned roughly.

The churlish tones were so unlike Tim that Sara looked up at him in some amazement. He was staring down at her with a strange, *awakened* expression in his eyes; his face was very white and his mouth working.

With a sudden apprehension of what was impending, she sprang up, stretching out her hand as though to ward it off.

"No--no, Tim. It isn't--don't say it's that----"

He caught her hand and held it between both his.

"But it *is* that," he said, speaking very fast, the serenity of his face all broken up by the surge of emotion that had gripped him. "It is that. I love you. I didn't know it till you spoke of going away. Sara--"

"Oh, I'm sorry, I'm sorry!" She broke in hastily. "Don't say any more, Tim--please don't!"

In the silence that followed the two young faces peered at each other--the one desperate with love, the other full of infinite regret and pleading.

At last--

"It's no use, then?" said Tim dully. "You don't care?"

"I'm afraid I don't--not like that. I thought we were friends--just friends, Tim," she urged.

Tim lifted his head, and she saw that somehow, in the last few minutes, he had grown suddenly older. His gay, smiling mouth had set itself sternly; the beautiful boyish face had become a man's.

"I thought so, too," he said gently. "But I know now that what I feel for you isn't friendship. It's"--with a short, grim laugh--"something much more than that. Tell me, Sara--will there ever be any chance for me?"

She hesitated. She was so genuinely fond of him that she hated to give him pain. Looking at him, standing before her in his splendid young manhood, she wondered irritably why she *didn't* love him. He was pre-eminently loveable.

He caught eagerly at her hesitation.

"Don't answer me now!" he said swiftly. "I'll wait--give me a chance. I can't take no . . . I won't take it!" he went on masterfully. "I love you!" Impetuously he slipped his strong young arms about her and kissed her on the mouth.

The previous moment she had been all softness and regret, but now, at the sudden passion in his voice, something within her recoiled violently, repudiating the claim his love had made upon her.

Sara was the last woman in the world to be taken by storm. She was too individual, her sense of personal independence too strongly developed, for her ever to be swept off her feet by a passion to which her own heart offered no response. Instead, it roused her to a definite consciousness of opposition, and she drew herself away from Tim's eager arms with a decision there was no mistaking.

"I'm sorry, Tim," she said quietly. "But it's no good pretending I'm in love with you. I'm not."

He looked at her with moody, dissatisfied eyes.

"I've spoken too soon," he said. "I should have waited. Only I was afraid."

"Afraid?"

"Yes." He spoke uncertainly. "I've had a feeling that if I let you go, you'll meet some man down there, at Monkshaven, who'll want to marry you . . . And I shall lose you! . . . Oh, Sara! I don't ask you to say you love me--yet. Say that you'll marry me . . . I'd teach you the rest--you'd learn to love me."

But that fierce, unpremeditated kiss--the first lover's kiss that she had known--had endowed her with a sudden clarity of vision.

"No," she answered steadily. "I don't know much about love, Tim, but I'm very sure it's no use trying to manufacture it to order, and--listen, Tim, dear," the pain in his face making her suddenly all tenderness again--"if I married you, and afterwards you *couldn't* teach me as you think you could, we should only be wretched together."

"I could never be wretched if you were my wife," he answered doggedly. "I've love enough for two."

She shook her head.

"No, Tim. Don't let's spoil a good friendship by turning it into a one-sided love-affair."

He smiled rather grimly.

"I'm afraid it's too late to prevent that," he said drily. "But I won't worry you any more now, dear. Only--I'm not going to accept your answer as final."

"I wish you would," she urged.

He looked at her curiously. "No man who loves you, Sara, is going to give you up very easily," he averred. Then, after a moment: "you'll let me write to you sometimes?"

She nodded soberly.

"Yes--but not love-letters, Tim."

"No--not love-letters."

He lifted her hands and kissed first one and then the other. Then, with his head well up and his shoulders squared, he went away.

But the sea-blue eyes that had been wont to look out on the world so gaily had suddenly lost their care-free bravery. They were the eyes of a man who has looked for the first time into the radiant, sorrowful face of Love, and read therein all the possibilities--the glory and the pain and the supreme happiness--which Love holds.

And Sara, standing alone and regretful that the friend had been lost in the lover, never guessed that Tim's love was a thread which was destined to cross and re-cross those other threads held by the fingers of Fate until it had tangled the whole fabric of her life.

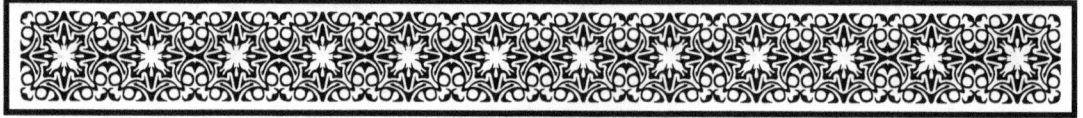

CHAPTER V
THE MAN IN THE TRAIN

Oldhampton! Oldhampton! Change here for Motchley and Monkshaven!" It was with a sigh of relief that Sara, in obedience to the warning raucously intoned by a hurrying porter, vacated her seat in the railway compartment in which she had travelled from Fallowdene. Her companions on the journey had been an elderly spinster and her maid, and as the former had insisted upon the exclusion of every breath of outside air, Sara felt half-suffocated by the time they ran into Oldhampton Junction. The Monkshaven train was already standing in the station, and, commissioning a porter to transfer her luggage, she sauntered leisurely along the platform, searching vainly for an empty compartment, where the regulation of the supply of oxygen would not depend upon the caprice of an old maid.

The train appeared to be very full, but at last she espied a first-class smoking carriage which boasted but a single occupant--a man in the far corner, half-hidden behind the newspaper he was holding--and, tipping her porter, she stepped into the compartment and busied herself bestowing her hand-baggage in the rack.

The man in the corner abruptly lowered his newspaper.

"This be a smoker," he remarked significantly.

Sara turned at the sound of his voice. The unwelcoming tones made it abundantly clear that the remainder of his thought ran: "And you've no business to get into it." A spark of amusement lit itself in her eyes.

"The railway company indicate as much on the window," she replied placidly, with a glance towards the *Smoking Carriage* label pasted against the pane.

There came no response, unless an irritated crackling of newspaper could be regarded as such--and the next moment, to the accompaniment of much banging of doors and a final shout of: "Stand away there!" the train began to move slowly out of the station.

Sara sat down with a sigh of relief that she had escaped her former travelling companions, with their unpleasant predilection for a vitiated atmosphere, and her thoughts wandered idly to the consideration of the man in the corner, to whom she was obviously an equally unwelcome fellow-passenger.

He had retired once more behind his newspaper, and practically all that was offered for her contemplation consisted of a pair of knee-breeches and well-cut leather leggings and two strong-looking, sun-tanned hands. These latter intrigued Sara considerably--their long, sensitive fingers and short, well-kept nails according curiously with their sunburnt suggestion of great physical strength and an outdoor life. She wished their owner would see fit to lower his newspaper once more, since her momentary glimpse of his face had supplied her with but little idea of his personality. And the hands, so full of contradictory suggestion, aroused her interest.

As though in response to her thoughts, the newspaper suddenly crackled down on to its owner's knees.

"I have every intention of smoking," he announced aggressively. "This is a smoking carriage."

Sara, supported by the recollection of a dainty little gold and enamel affair in her hand-bag, filled with some very special Russian cigarettes, smiled amiably.

"I know it is," she replied in unruffled tones. "That's why I got in. I, too, have every intention of smoking."

He stared at her in silence for a moment, then, without further comment, produced a pipe and tobacco pouch from the depths of a pocket, and proceeded to fill the former, carefully pressing down the tobacco with the tip of one of those slender, capable-looking fingers.

Sara observed him quickly. As he lounged there indolently in his corner, she was aware of a subtle combination of strength and fine tempering in the long, supple lines of his limbs--something that suggested the quality of steel, hard, yet pliant. He had a lean, hard-bitten face, tanned by exposure to the sun and wind, and the clean-shaven lips met with a curious suggestion of bitter reticence in their firm closing. His hair was brown--"plain brown" as Sara mentally characterized it--but it had a redeeming kink in it and the crispness of splendid vitality. The eyes beneath the straight, rather frowning brows were hazel, and, even in the brief space of time occupied by the inimical colloquy of a few moments ago, Sara had been struck by the peculiar intensity of their regard--an odd depth and brilliance only occasionally to be met with, and then preferably in those eyes which are a somewhat light grey in colour and ringed round the outer edge of the iris with a deeper tint.

The flare of a match roused her from her half-idle, half-interested contemplation of her fellow-passenger, and, as he lit his pipe, she was sharply conscious that his oddly luminous eyes were regarding her with a glint of irony in their depths.

Instantly she recalled his hostile reception of her entrance into the compartment, and the defiantly given explanation she had tendered in return.

Very deliberately she extracted her cigarette-case from her bag and selected a cigarette, only to discover that she had not supplied herself with a matchbox. She hunted assiduously amongst the assortment of odds and ends the bag contained, but in vain, and finally, a little nettled that her companion made no attempt to supply the obvious deficiency, she looked up to find that he was once more, to all appearances, completely absorbed in his newspaper.

Sara regarded him with indignation; in her own mind she was perfectly convinced that he was aware of her quandary and had no mind to help her out of it. Evidently he had not forgiven her intrusion into his solitude.

"Boor!" she ejaculated mentally. Then, aloud, and with considerable acerbity: "Could you oblige me with a match?"

With no show of alacrity, and with complete indifference of manner, he produced a matchbox and handed it to her, immediately reverting to his newspaper as though considerably bored by the interruption.

Sara flushed, and, having lit her cigarette, tendered him his matchbox with an icy little word of thanks.

Apparently, however, he was quite unashamed of his churlishness, for he accepted the box without troubling to raise his eyes from the page he was reading, and the remainder of the journey to Monkshaven was accomplished in an atmosphere that bristled with hostility.

As the train slowed up into the station, it became evident to Sara that Monkshaven was also the destination of her travelling companion, for he proceeded with great deliberation to fold up his newspaper and to hoist his suit-case down from the rack.

It did not seem to occur to him to proffer his service to Sara, who was struggling with her own hand-luggage, and the instant the train came to a standstill he opened the door of the compartment, stopped out on to the platform, and marched away.

A gleam of amusement crossed her face.

"I wonder who he is?" she reflected, as she followed in the wake of a porter in search of her trunks. "He certainly needs a lesson in manners."

Within herself she registered a vindictive vow that, should the circumstances of her residence in Monkshaven afford the opportunity, she would endeavour to give him one.

Monkshaven was but a tiny little station, and it was soon apparent that no conveyance of any kind had been sent to meet her.

"No, there would be none," opined the porter of whom she inquired. "Dr. Selwyn keeps naught but a little pony-trap, and he's most times using it himself. But there's a 'bus from the Cliff Hotel meets all trains, miss, and"--with pride--"there's a station keb."

In a few minutes Sara was the proud--and thankful--occupant of the "station keb," and, after bumping over the cobbles with which the station yard was paved, she found herself being driven in leisurely fashion through the high street of the little town, whilst her driver, sitting sideways on his box, indicated the points of interest with his whip as they went along.

Presently the cab turned out of the town and began the ascent of a steep hill, and as they climbed the winding road, Sara found that she could glimpse the sea, rippling greyly beyond the town, and tufted with little bunches of spume whipped into being by the keen March wind. The town itself spread out before her, an assemblage of red and grey tiled roofs sloping downwards to the curve of the bay, while, on the right, a bold promontory thrust itself into the sea, grimly resisting the perpetual onslaught of the wave. Through the waning light of the winter's afternoon, Sara could discern the outline of a house limned against the dark background of woods that crowned it. Linked to the jutting headland, a long range of sea-washed cliffs stretched as far as the eyes could reach.

"That be Monk's Cliff," vouchsafed the driver conversationally. "Bit of a lonesome place for folks to choose to live at, ain't it?"

"Who lives there?" asked Sara with interest.

"Gentleman of the name of Trent--queer kind of bloke he must be, too, if all's true they say of 'im. He's lived there a matter of ten years or more--lives by 'imself with just a man and his wife to do for 'im. Far End, they calls the 'ouse."

"Far End," repeated Sara. The name conveyed an odd sense of remoteness and inaccessibility. It seemed peculiarly appropriate to a house built thus on the very edge of the mainland.

Her eyes rested musingly on the bleak promontory. It would be a fit abode, she thought, for some recluse, determined to eschew the society of his fellow-men; here he could dwell, solitary and apart, surrounded on three sides by the grey, dividing sea, and protected on the fourth by the steep untempting climb that lay betwixt the town and the lonely house on the cliff.

"'Ere you are, miss. This is Dr. Selwyn's."

The voice of her Jehu roused her from her reflections to find that the cab had stopped in front of a white-painted wooden gate bearing the legend, "Sunnyside," painted in black letters across its topmost bar.

"I'll take the keb round to the stable-yard, miss; it'll be more convenient-like for the luggage," added the man, with a mildly disapproving glance towards the narrow tiled path leading from the gate to the house-door.

Sara nodded, and, having paid him his fare, made her way through the white gateway and along the path.

There seemed a curious absence of life about the place. No sound of voices broke the silence, and, although the front door stood invitingly open, there was no sign of any one hovering in the background ready to receive her.

Vaguely chilled--since, of course, they must be expecting her--she rang the bell. It clanged noisily through the house but failed to produce any more important result than the dislodging of some dust from a ledge above which the bell-wire ran. Sara watched it fall and lie on the floor in a little patch of fine, greyish powder.

The hall, of which the open door gave view, though of considerable dimensions, was poorly furnished. The wide expanse of colour-washed wall was broken only by a hat-stand, on which hung a large assortment of masculine hats and coats, all of them looking considerably the worse for wear, and by two straight-backed chairs placed with praiseworthy exactitude at equal distances apart from the afore-said rather overburdened piece of furniture. The floor was covered with linoleum of which the black and white chess-board pattern had long since retrogressed with usage into an uninspiring blur. A couple of threadbare rugs completed a somewhat depressing "interior."

Sara rang the bell a second time, on this occasion with an irritable force that produced clangour enough, one would have thought, to awaken the dead. It served, at all events, to arouse the living, for presently heavy footsteps could be heard descending the stairs, and, finally, a middle-aged maidservant, whose cap had obviously been assumed in haste, appeared, confronting Sara with an air of suspicion that seemed rather to suggest that she might have come after the spoons.

"The doctor's out," she announced somewhat truculently. Then, before Sara had time to formulate any reply, she added, a thought more graciously: "Maybe you're a stranger to these parts. Surgery hour's not till six o'clock."

She was evidently fully prepared for Sara to accept this as a dismissal, and looked considerably astonished when the latter queried meekly:

"Then can I see Miss Selwyn, please? I understand Mrs. Selwyn is an invalid."

"You're right there. The mistress isn't up for seeing visitors. And Miss Molly, she's not home--she's away to Oldhampton."

"But--but----" stammered Sara. "They're expecting me, surely? I'm Miss Tennant," she added by way of explanation.

"Miss Tennant! Sakes alive!" The woman threw up her hands, staring at Sara with an almost comic expression, halting midway between bewilderment and horror. "If that isn't just the way of them," she went on indignantly, "never mentioning that 'twas to-day you were coming--and no sheets aired to your bed and all! The master, he never so much as named it to me, nor Miss Molly neither. But please to come in, miss--" her outraged sense of hospitality infusing a certain limited cordiality into her tones.

The woman led the way into a sitting-room that opened off the hall, standing aside for Sara to pass in, then, muttering half-inaudibly, "You'll be liking a cup of tea, I expect," she disappeared into the back regions of the house, whence a distant clattering of china shortly gave indication that the proffered refreshment was in course of preparation.

Sara seated herself in a somewhat battered armchair and proceeded to take stock of the room in which she found herself. It tallied accurately with what the hall had led her to expect. Most of the furniture had been good of its kind at one time, but it was now all reduced to a drab level of shabbiness. There were a few genuine antiques amongst it--a couple of camel-backed Chippendale chairs, a grandfather's clock, and some fine old bits of silver--which Sara's eye, accustomed to the rare and beautiful furnishings of Barrow Court, singled out at once from the olla podrida of incongruous modern stuff. These alone had survived the general condition of disrepair; but, even so, the silver had a neglected appearance and stood badly in need of cleaning.

This latter criticism might have been leveled with equal justice at almost everything in the room, and Sara, mindful of her reception, reflected that in such an oddly conducted household, where the advent of an expected, and obviously much-needed, paying guest could be completely overlooked, it was hardly probable that smaller details of house-management would receive their meed of attention.

Instead of depressing her, however, the forlorn aspect of the room assisted to raise her spirits. It looked as though there might very well be a niche in such a household that she could fill. Mentally she proceeded to make a tour of the room, duster in hand, and she had just reached the point where, in imagination, she was about to place a great bowl of flowers in the middle desert of the table, when the elderly Abigail re-appeared and dumped a tea-tray down in front of her.

Sara made a wry face over the tea. It tasted flat, and she could well imagine the long-boiling kettle from which the water with which it had been made was poured.

"I'm sure that tea's beastly!"

A masculine voice sounded abruptly from the doorway, and, looking up, Sara beheld a tall, eager-faced man, wearing a loose shabby coat and carrying in one hand a professional-looking doctor's bag. The bag, however, was the only professional-looking thing about him. For the rest, he might have been taken to be either an impoverished country squire and sportsman, or a Roman Catholic dignitary, according to whether you assessed him by his broad, well-knit figure and weather-beaten complexion, puckered with wrinkles born of jolly laughter, or by the somewhat austere and controlled set of his mouth and by the ardent luminous grey eyes, with their touch of the visionary and fanatic.

Sara set down her cup hastily.

"And I'm sure you're Dr. Selwyn," she said, a flicker of amusement at his unconventional greeting in her voice.

"Right!" he answered, shaking hands. "How are you, Miss Tennant? It was plucky of you to decide to risk us after all, and I hope--" with a slight grimace--"you won't find we are any worse than I depicted. I was very sorry I had to be out when you came," he went on genially, "but I expect Molly has looked after you all right? By the way"--glancing round him in some perplexity--"where *is* Molly?"

"I understood," replied Sara tranquilly, "that she had gone in to Oldhampton."

Dr. Selwyn's expression was not unlike that of a puppy caught in the unlawful possession of his master's slipper.

"What did I warn you?" he exclaimed with a rueful laugh. "We're quite a hopeless household, I'm afraid. And Molly's the most absent-minded of beings. I expect she has clean forgotten that you were coming to-day. She's by way of being an artist--art-student, rather"--correcting himself with a smile. "You know the kind of thing--black carpets and Futurist colour schemes in dress. So you must try and forgive her. She's only seventeen. But Jane--I hope Jane did the honours properly? She is our stand-by in all emergencies."

Sara's eyes danced.

"I'm afraid I came upon Jane entirely in the light of an unpleasant surprise," she responded mildly.

"What! Do you mean to say she wasn't prepared for you? Oh, but this is scandalous! What must you think of us all?" he strode across the room and pealed the bell, and, when Jane appeared in answer to the summons, demanded wrathfully why nothing was in readiness for Miss Tennant's arrival.

Jane surveyed him with the immovable calm of the old family servant, her arms akimbo.

"And how should it be?" she wanted to know. "Seeing that neither you nor Miss Molly named it to me that the young lady was coming to-day?"

"But I asked Miss Molly to make arrangements," protested Selwyn feebly.

"And did you expect her to do so, sir, may I ask?" inquired Jane with withering scorn.

"Do you mean to tell me that Miss Molly gave you no orders about preparing a room?" countered the doctor, skillfully avoiding the point raised?

"No, sir, she didn't. And if I'm kep' here talking much longer, there won't *be*

one prepared, neither! 'Tis no use crying over spilt milk. Let me get on with the air-
ing of my sheets, and do you talk to the young lady whiles I see to it."

And Jane departed forthwith about her business.

"Jane Crab," observed Selwyn, twinkling, "has been with us five-and-twenty
years. I had better do as she tells me." He threw a doleful glance at the unappetizing
tea in Sara's cup. "I positively dare not order you fresh tea--in the circumstances.
Jane would probably retaliate with an ultimatum involving a rigid choice between
tea and the preparation of your room, accompanied by a pithy summary of the ca-
pabilities of one pair of hands."

"Wouldn't you like some tea yourself?" hazarded Sara.

"I should--very much. But I see no prospect of getting any while Jane maintains
her present attitude of mind."

"Then--if you will show me the kitchen--*I'll* make some," announced Sara
valiantly.

Selwyn regarded her with a pitying smile.

"You don't know Jane," he said. "Trespassers in the kitchen are not--welcomed."

"And Jane doesn't know *me*," replied Sara firmly.

"On your own head be it, then," retorted the doctor, and led the way to the
sacrosanct domain presided over by Jane Crab.

How Sara managed it Selwyn never knew, but she contrived to invade Jane's
kitchen and perform the office of tea-making without offending her in the very
least. Nay, more, by some occult process known only to herself, she succeeded in
winning Jane's capacious heart, and from that moment onwards, the autocrat of the
kitchen became her devoted satellite; and later, when Sara started to make drastic
changes in the slip-shod arrangements of the house, her most willing ally.

"Miss Tennant's the only body in the place as has got some sense in her head,"
she was heard to observe on more than one occasion.

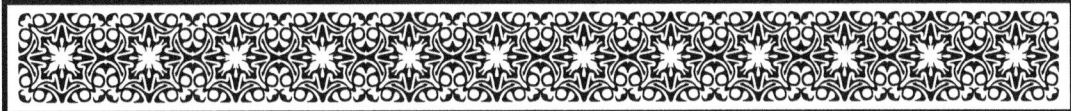

CHAPTER VI
THE SKELETON IN SELWYN'S CUPBOARD

After tea, Selwyn escorted Sara upstairs and introduced her to his wife. Mrs. Selwyn was a slender, colourless woman, possessing the remnants of what must at one time have been an ineffective kind of prettiness. She was a determinedly chronic invalid, and rarely left the rooms which had been set aside for her use to join the other members of the family downstairs.

"The stairs try my heart, you see," she told Sara, with the martyred air peculiar to the hypochondriac--the genuine sufferer rarely has it. "It is, of course, a great deprivation to me, and I don't think either Dick"--with an inimical glance at her husband--"or Molly come up to see me as often as they might. Stairs are no difficulty to *them*."

Selwyn, who invariably ran up to see his wife immediately on his return from no matter how long or how tiring a round of professional visits, bit his lip.

"I come as often as I can, Minnie," he said patiently. "You must remember my time is not my own."

"No, dear, of course not. And I expect that outside patients are much more interesting to visit than one's own wife," with a disagreeable little laugh.

"They mean bread-and-butter, anyway," said Selwyn bluntly.

"Of course they do." She turned to Sara. "Dick always thinks in terms of bread-and-butter, Miss Tennant," she said sneeringly. "But money means little enough to any one with my poor health. Beyond procuring me a few alleviations, there is nothing it can do for me."

Sara was privately of the opinion that it had done a good deal for her. Looking round the luxuriously furnished room with its blazing fire, and then at Mrs. Selwyn herself, elegantly clad in a rest-gown of rich silk, she could better understand the poverty-stricken appearance of the rest of the house, Dick's shabby clothes, and his willingness to receive a paying guest whose contribution towards the housekeeping might augment his slender income.

Here, then, was where his hard-earned guineas went--to keep in luxury this petulant, complaining woman whose entire thoughts were centred about her own bodily comfort, and whom Patrick Lovell, with his lucid recognition of values, would have contemptuously described as "a parasite woman, m'dear--the kind of female I've no use for."

"Oh, Dick"--Mrs. Selwyn had been turning over the pages of a price-list that was lying on her knee--"I see the World's Store have just brought out a new kind of adjustable reading-table. It's a much lighter make than the one I have. I think I should find it easier to use."

Selwyn's face clouded.

"How much does it cost, dear?" he asked nervously. "These mechanical contrivances are very expensive, you know."

"Oh, this one isn't. It's only five guineas."

"Five guineas is rather a lot of money, Minnie," he said gravely. "Couldn't you manage with the table you have for a bit longer?"

Mrs. Selwyn tossed the price-list pettishly on to the floor.

"Of, of course!" she declared. "That's always the way. 'Can't I manage with what I have? Can't I make do with this, that, and the other?' I believe you grudge every penny you spend on me!" she wound up acrimoniously.

A dull red crept into Selwyn's face.

"You know it's not that, Minnie," he replied in a painfully controlled voice. "It's simply that I **can't afford** these things. I give you everything I can. If I were only a rich man, you should have everything you want."

"Perhaps if you were to work a little more intelligently you'd make more money," she retorted. "If only you'd keep your brains for the use of people who can **pay**--and pay well--I shouldn't be deprived of every little comfort I ask for! Instead of that, you've got half the poor of Monkshaven on your hands--and if you think they can't afford to pay, you simply don't send in a bill. Oh, *I* know!"--sitting up excitedly in her chair, a patch of angry scarlet staining each cheek--"I hear what goes on--even shut away from the world as I am. It's just to curry popularity--you get all the praise, and I suffer for it! *I* have to go without what I want--"

"Oh, hush! Hush!" Selwyn tried ineffectually to stem the torrent of complaint.

"No, I won't hush! It's 'Doctor Dick this,' and 'Doctor Dick that'--oh, yes, you see, I know their name for you, these slum patients of yours!--but it's Doctor Dick's wife who really foots the bills--by going without what she needs!"

"Minnie, be quiet!" Selwyn broke in sternly. "Remember Miss Tennant is present."

But she had got beyond the stage when the presence of a third person, even that of an absolute stranger, could be depended upon to exercise any restraining effect.

"Well, since Miss Tenant's going to live here, the sooner she knows how things stand the better! She won't be here long without seeing how I'm treated"--her voice rising hysterically--"set on one side, and denied even the few small pleasures my health permits----"

She broke off in a storm of angry weeping, and Sara retreated hastily from the room, leaving husband and wife alone together.

She had barely regained the shabby sitting-room when the front door opened and closed with a bang, and a gay voice could be heard calling--

"Jane! Jane! Come here, my pretty Jane! I've brought home some shrimps for tea!"

"Hold your noise, Miss Molly, now do!"

Sara could hear Jane's admonitory whisper, and there followed a murmured colloquy, punctuated by exclamations and gusts of young laughter, calling forth renewed remonstrance from Jane, and then the door of the room was flung open, and Molly Selwyn sailed in and overwhelmed Sara with apologies for her reception, or rather, for the lack of it. She was quite charming in her penitence, waving dimpled, deprecating hands, and appealing to Sara with a pair of liquid, disarming, golden-brown eyes that earned her forgiveness on the spot.

She was a statuesque young creature, compact of large, soft, gracious curves and swaying movements--with her nimbus of pale golden hair, and curiously floating, undulating walk, rather reminding one of a stray goddess. Always untidy with hooks lacking at important junctures, and the trimmings of her hats usually pinned on with a casualness that occasionally resulted in their deserting the hat altogether, she could still never be other than delightful and irresistibly desirable to look upon.

Her red, curving mouth of a child, cleft chin, and dimpled, tapering hands all promised a certain yieldingness of disposition--a tendency to take always the line of least resistance--but it was a charming, appealing kind of frailty which most people--the sterner sex, certainly--would be very ready to condone.

It is a wonderful thing to be young. Molly poured herself out a cup of hideously stewed tea and drank it joyously to an accompaniment of shrimps and bread-and-butter, and when Sara uttered a mild protest, she only laughed and declared that it was a wholesome and digestible diet compared with some of the "studio teas" perpetrated by the artists' colony at Oldhampton, of which she was a member.

She chattered away gaily to Sara, giving her vivacious thumb-nail portraits of her future neighbours--the people Selwyn had described as being "much nicer than ourselves."

"The Herricks and Audrey Maynard are our most intimate friends--I'm sure you'll adore them. Mrs. Maynard is a widow, and if she weren't so frightfully rich, Monkshaven would be perennially shocked at her. She is ultra-fashionable, and smokes whenever she chooses, and swears when ordinary language fails her--all of which things, of course, are anathema to the select circles of Monkshaven. But then she's a millionaire's widow, so instead of giving her the cold shoulder, every one gushes round her and declares 'Mrs. Maynard is such a thoroughly *modern* type, you know!'"--Molly mimicked the sugar-and-vinegar accents of the critics to perfection--"and privately Audrey shouts with laughter at them, while publicly she continues to shock them for the sheer joy of the thing."

"And who are the Herricks?" asked Sara, smiling. "Married people?"

"No." Molly shook her head. "Miles is a bachelor who lives with a maiden aunt--Miss Lavinia. Or, rather, she lives with him and housekeeps for him. 'The Lavender Lady,' I always call her, because she's one of those delightful old-fashioned people who remind one of dimity curtains, and pot-pourri, and little muslin bags of lavender. Miles is a perfect pet, but he's lame, poor dear."

Sara waited with a curious eagerness for any description which might seem to fit her recent fellow-traveller, but none came, and at last she threw out a question in the hope of eliciting his name.

"He was horribly ungracious and rude," she added, "and yet he didn't look in the least the sort of man who would be like that. There was no lack of breeding about him. He was just deliberately snubby--as though I had no right to exist on the same planet with him--anyway"--laughing--"not in the same railway compartment."

Molly nodded sagely.

"I believe I know whom you mean. Was he a lean, brown, grim-looking individual, with the kind of eyes that almost make you jump when they look at you suddenly?"

"That certainly describes them," admitted Sara, smiling faintly.

"Then it was the Hermit of Far End," announced Molly.

"The Hermit of Far End?"

"Yes. He's a queer, silent man who lives all by himself at a house built almost on the edge of Monk's Cliff--you must have seen it as you drove up?"

"Oh!" exclaimed Sara, with sudden enlightenment. "Then his name is Trent. The cabman presented me with that information," she added, in answer to Molly's look of surprise.

"Yes--Garth Trent. It's rather an odd name--sounds like a railway collision, doesn't it? But it suits him somehow"--reflectively.

"Have you met him?" prompted Sara. It was odd how definite an interest her brief encounter with him had aroused in her.

"Yes--once. He treated me"--giggling delightedly--"rather as if I *wasn't there*! At least"--reminiscently--"he tried to."

"It doesn't sound as though he had succeeded?" suggested Sara, amused.

Molly looked at her solemnly.

"He told some one afterwards--Miles Herrick, the only man he ever speaks to, I think, without compulsion--that I was 'the Delilah type of woman, and ought to have been strangled at birth.'"

"He must be a charming person," commented Sara ironically.

"Oh, he's a woman-hater--in fact, I believe he has a grudge against the world in general, but woman in particular. I expect"--shrewdly--"he's been crossed in love."

At this moment Selwyn re-entered the room, his grave face clearing a little as he caught sight of his daughter.

"Hullo, Molly mine! Got back, then?" he said, smiling. "Have you made your peace with Miss Tennant, you scatterbrained young woman?"

"It's a hereditary taint, Dad--don't blame *me*!" retorted Molly with lazy impudence, pulling his head down and kissing him on the top of his ruffled hair.

Selwyn grinned.

"I pass," he submitted. "And who is it that's been crossed in love?"

"The Hermit of Far End."

"Oh"--turning to Sara--"so you have been discussing our local enigma?"

"Yes. I fancy I must have travelled down with him from Oldhampton. He seemed rather a boorish individual."

"He would be. He doesn't like women."

"Monk's Cliff would appear to be an appropriate habitation for him, then," commented Sara tartly.

They all laughed, and presently Selwyn suggested that his daughter should run up and see her mother.

"She'll be hurt if you don't go up, kiddy," he said. "And try and be very nice to her--she's a little tired and upset to-day."

When she had left the room he turned to Sara, a curious blending of proud reluctance and regret in his eyes.

"I'm so sorry, Miss Tennant," he said simply, "that you should have seen our worst side so soon after your arrival. You--you must try and pardon it--"

"Oh, please, please don't apologize," broke in Sara hastily. "I'm so sorry I happened to be there just then. It was horrible for you."

He smiled at her wistfully.

"It's very kind of you to take it like that," he said. "After all"--frankly--"you could not have remained with us very long without finding out our particular skeleton in the cupboard. My wife's state of health--or, rather, what she believes to be her state of health--is a great grief to me. I've tried in every way to convince her that she is not really so delicate as she imagines, but I've failed utterly."

Now that the ice was broken, he seemed to find relief in pouring out the pitiful little tragedy of his home life.

"She is comparatively young, you know, Miss Tennant--only thirty-seven, and she willfully leads the life of a confirmed invalid. It has grown upon her gradually, this absorption in her health, and now, practically speaking, Molly has no mother and I no wife."

"Oh, Doctor Dick"--the little nickname, that had its origin in his slum patients' simple affection for the man who tended them, came instinctively from her lips. It seemed, somehow, to fit itself to the big, kindly man with the sternly rugged face and eyes of a saint. "Oh, Doctor Dick, I'm so sorry--so very sorry!"

Perhaps something in the dainty, well-groomed air of the woman beside him helped to accentuate the neglected appearance of the room, for he looked round in an irritated kind of way, as though all at once conscious of its deficiencies.

"And this--this, too," he muttered. "There's no one at the helm. . . . The truth is, I ought never to have let you come here."

Sara shook her head.

"I've very glad I came," she said simply. "I think I'm going to be very happy here."

"You've got grit," he replied quietly. "You'd make a success of your life any-where. I wish"--thoughtfully--"Molly had a little of that same quality. Sometimes"--a worried frown gathered on his face--"I get afraid for Molly. She's such a child . . . and no mother to hold the reins."

"Doctor Dick, would you consider it impertinent if--if I laid my hands on the reins--just now and then?"

He whirled round, his eyes shining with gratitude.

"Impertinent! I should be illimitably thankful! You can see how things are--I am compelled to be out all my time, my wife hardly ever leaves her own rooms, and Molly and the house affairs just get along as best they can."

"Then," said Sara, smiling, "I shall put my finger in the pie. I've--I've no one to look after now, since Uncle Patrick died," she added. "I think, Doctor Dick, I've found my job."

"It's absurd!" he exclaimed, regarding her with unfeigned delight. "Here you come along, prepared, no doubt, to be treated as a 'guest,' and the first thing I do is to shovel half my troubles on to your shoulders. It's absurd--disgraceful! . . . But it's amazingly good!" He held out his hand, and as Sara's slim fingers slid into his big palm, he muttered a trifle huskily: "God bless you for it, my dear!"

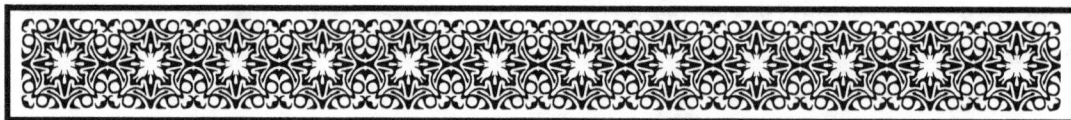

CHAPTER VII
TRESPASS

Sara stood on the great headland known as Monk's Cliff, watching with delight the white-topped billows hurling themselves against its mighty base, only to break in a baulked fury of thunder and upflung spray.

She had climbed the steep ascent thither on more than one day of storm and bluster, reveling in the buffeting of the gale and in the pungent tang of brine from the spray-drenched air. The cry of the wind, shrieking along the face of the sea-bitten cliff, reminded her of the scream of the hurricane as it tore through the pine-woods at Barrow--shaking their giant tops hither and thither as easily as a child's finger might shake a Canterbury bell.

Something wild and untamed within her responded to the savage movement of the scene, and she stood for a long time watching the expanse of restless, wind-tossed waters, before turning reluctantly in the direction of home. If for nothing else than for this gift of glorious sea and cliff, she felt she could be content to pitch her tent in Monkshaven indefinitely.

Her way led past Far End, the solitary house perched on the sloping side of the headland, and, as she approached, she became aware of a curious change of character in the sound of the wind. She was sheltered now from its fiercest onslaught, and it seemed to her that it rose and fell, moaning in strange, broken cadences, almost like the singing of a violin.

She paused a moment, thinking at first that this was due to the wind's whining through some narrow passage betwixt the outbuildings of the house, then, as the chromatic wailing broke suddenly into vibrating harmonies, she realized that some one actually *was* playing the violin, and playing it remarkably well, too.

Instinctively she yielded to the fascination of it, and, drawing nearer to the house, leaned against a sheltered wall, all her senses subordinate to that of hearing.

Whoever the musician might be, he was a thorough master of his instrument, and Sara listened with delight, recognizing some of the haunting melodies of the wild Russian music which he was playing--music that even in its moments of delirious joy seemed to hold always an underlying *bourdon* of tragedy and despair.

"Hi, there!"

She started violently. Entirely absorbed in the music, she had failed to observe a man, dressed in the style of an indoor servant, who had appeared in the doorway of one of the outbuildings and who now addressed her in peremptory tones.

"Hi, there! Don't you know you're trespassing?"

Jerked suddenly out of her dreamy enjoyment, Sara looked round vaguely.

"I didn't know that Monk's Cliff was private property," she said after a pause.

"Nor is it, that I know of. But you're on the Far End estate now--this is a private road," replied the man disagreeably. "You'll please to take yourself off."

A faint flush of indignation crept up under the warm pallor of Sara's skin. Then, a sudden thought striking her, she asked--

"Who is that playing the violin?"

Mentally she envisioned a pair of sensitive, virile hands, lean and brown, with the short, well-kept nails that any violinist needs must have--the contradictory hands which had aroused her interest on the journey to Monkshaven.

"I don't hear no one playing," replied the man stolidly. She felt certain he was lying, but he gave her no opportunity for further interrogation, for he continued briskly--

"Come now, miss, please to move off from here. Trespassers aren't allowed."

Sara spoke with a quiet air of dignity.

"Certainly I'll go," she said. "I'm sorry. I had no idea that I was trespassing."

The man's truculent manner softened, as, with the intuition of his kind, he recognized in the composed little apology the utterance of one of his "betters."

"Beggin' your pardon, miss," he said, with a considerable accession of civility, "but it's as much as my place is worth to allow a trespasser here on Far End."

Sara nodded.

"You're perfectly right to obey orders," she said, and bending her steps towards the public road from which she had strayed to listen to the unseen musician, she made her way homewards.

"Your mysterious 'Hermit' is nothing if not thorough," she told Doctor Dick and Molly on her return. "I trespassed on to the Far End property to-day, and was ignominiously ordered off by a rather aggressive person, who, I suppose, is Mr. Trent's servant."

"That would be Judson," nodded Selwyn. "I've attended him once or twice professionally. The fellow's all right, but he's under strict orders, I believe, to allow no trespassers."

"So it seems," returned Sara. "By the way, who is the violinist at Far End? Is it the 'Hermit' himself?"

"It's rumoured that he does play," said Molly. "But no one has ever been privileged to hear him."

"Their loss, then," commented Sara shortly. "I should say he is a magnificent performer."

Molly nodded, an expression of impish amusement in her eyes.

"On the sole occasion I met him, I asked him why no one was ever allowed to hear him play," she said, chuckling. "I even suggested that he might contribute a solo to the charity concert we were getting up at the time!"

"And what did he say?" asked Sara, smiling.

"Told me that there was no need for a man to exhibit his soul to the public! So I asked him what he meant, and he said that if I understood anything about music I would know, and that if I didn't, it was a waste of his time trying to explain. Do *you* know what he meant?"

"Yes," said Sara slowly, "I think I do." And recalling the passionate appeal and sadness of the music she had heard that afternoon, she was conscious of a sudden quick sense of pity for the solitary hermit of Far End. He was *afraid*--afraid to play to any one, lest he should reveal some inward bitterness of his soul to those who listened!

The following day, Molly carried Sara off to Rose Cottage to make the acquaintance of "the Lavender Lady" and her nephew.

Miss Herrick--or Miss Lavinia, as she was invariably addressed--looked exactly as though she had just stepped out of the early part of last century. She wore a gown of some soft, silky material, sprigged with heliotrope, and round her neck a fichu of cobwebby lace, fastened at the breast with a cameo brooch of old Italian workmanship. A coquettish little lace cap adorned the silver-grey hair, and the face beneath the cap was just what you would have expected to find it--soft and very gentle, its porcelain pink and white a little faded, the pretty old eyes a misty, lavender blue.

She was alone when the two girls arrived, and greeted Sara with a humorous little smile.

"How kind of you to come, Miss Tennant! We've been all agog to meet you, Miles and I. In a tiny place like Monkshaven, you see, every one knows every one else's business, so of course we have been hearing of you constantly."

"Then you might have come to Sunnyside to investigate me personally," replied Sara, smiling back.

Miss Lavinia's face sobered suddenly, a shadow falling across her kind old eyes.

"Miles is--rather difficult about calling," she said hesitatingly. "You will understand--his lameness makes him a little self-conscious with strangers," she explained.

Sara looked distressed.

"Oh! Perhaps it would have been better if I had not come?" she suggested hastily. "Shall I run away and leave Molly here?"

Miss Lavinia flushed rose-pink.

"My dear, I hope Miles knows how to welcome a guest in his own house as befits a Herrick," she said, with a delicious little air of old-world dignity. "Indeed, it is an excellent thing for him to be dragged out of his shell. Only, please--will you remember?--treat him exactly as though he were not lame--never try to help him in any way. It is that which hurts him so badly--when people make allowances for his lameness. Just ignore it."

Sara nodded. She could understand that instinctive man's pride which recoiled from any tolerant recognition of a physical handicap.

"Was his lameness caused by an accident?" she asked.

"It came through a very splendid deed." Little Miss Lavinia's eyes glowed as she spoke. "He stopped a pair of runaway carriage-horses. They had taken fright at a motor-lorry, and, when they bolted, the coachman was thrown from the box, so that it looked as if nothing could save the occupants of the carriage. Miles flung himself at the horses' heads, and although, of course, he could not actually stop them single-handed, he so impeded their progress that a second man, who sprang forward to help, was able to bring them to a standstill."

"How plucky of him!" exclaimed Sara warmly. "You must be very proud of your nephew, Miss Lavinia!"

"She is," interpolated Molly affectionately. "Aren't you, dear Lavender Lady?"

Miss Lavinia smiled a trifle wistfully.

"Ah! My dear," she said sadly, "splendid things are done at such a cost, and when they are over we are apt to forget the splendour and remember only the heavy price. . . . My poor Miles was horribly injured--he had been dragged for yards, clinging to the horses' bridles--and for weeks we were not even sure if he would live. He has lived--but he will walk lame to the end of his life."

The little instinctive silence which followed was broken by the sound of voices in the hall outside, and, a minute later, Miles Herrick himself came into the room, escorting a very fashionably attired and distinctly attractive woman, whom Sara guessed at once to be Audrey Maynard.

She was not in the least pretty, but the narrowest of narrow skirts in vogue in the spring of 1914 made no secret of the fact that her figure was almost perfect. Her face was small and thin and inclined to be sallow, and beneath upward-slanting brows, to which art had undoubtedly added something, glimmered a pair of greenish-grey eyes, clear like rain. Nor was there any mistaking the fact that the rich copper-colour of the hair swathed beneath the smart little hat had come out of a bottle, and was in no way to be accredited to nature. It was small wonder that primitive Monkshaven stood aghast at such flagrant tampering with the obvious intentions of Providence.

But notwithstanding her up-to-date air of artificiality, there was something immensely likeable about Audrey Maynard. Behind it all, Sara sensed the real woman--clever, tactful, and generously warm-hearted.

Woman, when all is said and done, is frankly primitive in her instincts, and the desire to attract--with all its odd manifestations--is really but the outcome of her innate desire for home and a mate. It is this which lies at the root of most of her little vanities and weaknesses--and of all the big sacrifices of which she is capable as well. So she may be forgiven the former, and trusted to fall short but rarely of the latter when the crucial test comes.

"Miles and I have been--as usual--squabbling violently," announced Mrs. Maynard. "Sugar, please--lots of it," she added, as Herrick handed her her tea. "It was about the man who lives at Far End," she continued in reply to the Lavender Lady's smiling query. "Miles has been very irritating, and tried to smash all my suggested theories to bits. He insists that the Hermit is quite a commonplace, harmless young man--"

"He must be at least forty," interposed Herrick mildly.

Audrey frowned him into silence and continued--

"Now that's so dull, when half Monkshaven believes him to be a villain of the deepest dye, hiding from justice--or, possibly, a Bluebeard with an unhappy wife imprisoned somewhere in that weird old house of his."

Sara listened with undignified interest. It was strange how the enigmatical personality of the owner of Far End kept cropping up across her path.

"And what is your own opinion, Mrs. Maynard?" she asked.

Audrey flashed her a keen glance from her rain-clear eyes.

"I think he's a--sphinx," she said slowly.

"The Sphinx was a lady," objected Herrick pertinently.

"Mr. Trent's a masculine re-incarnation of her, then," retorted Mrs. Maynard, undefeated.

Herrick smiled tolerantly. He was a tall, slenderly built man, with whimsical brown eyes and the half-stern, half-sweet mouth of one who has been through the mill of physical pain.

"*Homme incompris*," he suggested lightly. "Give the fellow his due--he at least supplies the feminine half of Monkshaven with a topic of perennial interest."

Audrey took up the implied challenge with enthusiasm, and the two of them wrangled comfortably together till tea was over. Then she demanded a cigarette-- and another cushion--and finally sent Miles in search of some snapshots they had taken together and which he had developed since last they had met. She treated him exactly as though he suffered no handicap, demanding from him all the little services she would have asked from a man who was physically perfect.

Sara herself, accustomed to anticipating every need of Patrick Lovell's, would have been inclined to feel somewhat compunctious over allowing a lame man to wait upon her, yet, as she watched the eager way in which Miles responded to the visitor's behests, she realized that in reality Audrey was behaving with supreme tact. She let Miles feel himself a man as other men, not a mere "lame duck" to whom indulgence must needs be granted.

And once, when her hair just brushed his cheek, as he stooped over her to indicate some special point in one of the recently developed photos, Sara surprised a sudden ardent light in his quiet brown eyes that set her wondering whether possibly, the incessant sparring between Herrick and the lively, impulsive woman who shocked half Monkshaven, did not conceal something deeper than mere friendship.

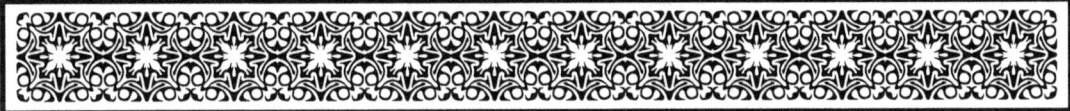

CHAPTER VIII
THE UNWILLING HOST

It was one of those surprisingly warm days, holding a foretaste of June's smiles, which March occasionally vouchsafes.

The sun blazed down out of a windless, cloudless sky, and Sara, making her way leisurely through the straggling woods that intervened betwixt the Selwyns' house and Monk's Cliff, felt the salt-laden air wafted against her face, as warmly mellow as though summer were already come.

Molly had gone to Oldhampton--since the artists' colony there would be certain to take advantage of this gift of a summer's day to arrange a sketching party, and, as the morning's post had brought Sara a letter from Elisabeth Durward which had occasioned her considerable turmoil of spirit, she had followed her natural bent by seeking the solitude of a lonely tramp in order to think the matter out.

From her earliest days at Barrow she had always carried the small tangles of childhood to a remote corner of the pine-woods for solution, and the habit had grown with her growth, so that now, when a rather bigger tangle presented itself, she turned instinctively to the solitude of the cliffs at Monkshaven, where the murmur of the sea was borne in her ears, plaintively reminiscent of the sound of the wind in her beloved pine trees.

Spring comes early in the sheltered, southern bay of Monkshaven, and already the bracken was sending up pushful little shoots of young green, curled like a baby's fist, while the primroses, bunched together in clusters, thrust peering faces impertinently above the green carpet of the woods. Sara stopped to pick a handful, tucking them into her belt. Then, emerging from the woods, she breasted the steep incline that led to the brow of the cliff.

A big boulder, half overgrown with moss and lichen, offered a tempting resting-place, and flinging herself down on the yielding turf beside it, she leaned back and drew out Elisabeth's letter.

She had sometimes wondered whether Elisabeth had any suspicion of the fact that, before leaving Barrow, she had refused to marry Tim. The friendship and understanding between mother and son was so deep that it was very possible that Tim had taken her into his confidence. And even if he had not, the eyesight of love is extraordinarily keen, and Elisabeth would almost inevitably have divined that something was amiss with his happiness.

If this were so, as Sara admitted to herself with a wry smile, there was little doubt that she would look askance at the woman who had had the temerity to refuse her beautiful Tim!

And now, although her letter contained no definite allusion to the matter, reading between the lines, the conviction was borne in upon Sara that Elisabeth knew all that there was to know, and had ranged herself, heart and soul, on the side of her son.

It was obvious that she thought of the whole world in terms of Tim, and, had she been a different type of woman, the simile of a hen with one chick would have occurred to Sara's mind.

But there was nothing in the least hen-like about Elisabeth Durward. Only, whenever Tim came near her, her face, with its strangely inscrutable eyes, would irradiate with a sudden warmth and tenderness of emotion that was akin to the exquisite rapture of a lover when the beloved is near. To Sara, there seemed something a little frightening--almost terrible--in her intense devotion to Tim.

The letter itself was charmingly written--expressing the hope that Sara was happy and comfortable at Monkshaven, recalling their pleasant time at Barrow together, and looking forward to other future visits from her--"*which would be a fulfillment of happiness to us all*."

It was this last sentence, combined with one or two other phrases into which much or little meaning might equally as easily be read, which had aroused in Sara a certain uneasy instinct of apprehension. Dimly she sensed a vague influence at work to strengthen the ties that bound her to Barrow, and to all that Barrow signified.

She faced the question with characteristic frankness. Tim had his own place in her heart--secure and unassailable. But it was not the place in that sacred inner temple which is reserved for the one man, and she recognized this with a limpid clearness of perception rather uncommon in a girl of twenty. She also recognized that it was within the bounds of possibility that the one man might never come to claim that place, and that, if she gave Tim the answer he so ardently desired, they would quite probably rub along together as well as most married folk--better, perhaps, than a good many. But she was very sure that she never intended to desecrate that inner temple by any lesser substitute for love.

Thus she reasoned, with the untried confidence of youth, which is so pathetically certain of itself and of its ultimate power to hold to its ideals, ignorant of the overpowering influences which may develop to push a man or woman this way or that, or of the pain that may turn clear, definite thought into a welter of blind anguish, when the soul in its agony snatches at any anodyne, true or false, which may seem to promise relief.

A little irritably she folded up Elisabeth's letter. It was disquieting in some ways--she could not quite explain why--and just now she felt averse to wrestling with disturbing ideas. She only wanted to lie still, basking in the tranquil peace of the afternoon, and listen to the murmuring voice of the sea.

She closed her eyes indolently, and presently, lulled by the drowsy rhythm of the waves breaking at the foot of the cliff, she fell asleep.

She woke with a start. An ominous drop of rain had splashed down on to her cheek, and she sat up, broad awake in an instant and shivering a little. It had turned much colder, and a wind had risen which whispered round her of coming storm, while the blue sky of an hour ago was hidden by heavy, platinum-coloured clouds massing up from the south.

Another and another raindrop fell, and, obeying their warning, Sara sprang up and bent her steps in the direction of home. But she was too late to avoid the storm which had been brewing, and before she had gone a hundred yards it had begun to break in drifting scurries of rain, driven before the wind.

She hurried on, hoping to gain the shelter of the woods before the threatened deluge, but within ten minutes of the first heralding drops it was upon her--a torrent of blinding rain, sweeping across the upland like a wet sheet.

She looked about her desperately, in search of cover, and perceiving, on the further side of a low stone wall, what she took to be a wooden shelter for cattle, she quickened her steps to a run, and, nimbly vaulting the wall, fled headlong into it.

It was not, however, the cattle shed she had supposed it, but a roughly constructed summer-house, open on one side to the four winds of heaven and with a wooden seat running round the remaining three.

Sara guessed immediately that she must have trespassed again on the Far End property, but reflecting that neither its owner nor his lynx-eyed servant was likely to be abroad in such a downpour as this, and that, even if they were, and chanced to discover her, they could hardly object to her taking refuge in this outlying shelter, she shook the rain from her skirts and sat down to await the lifting of the storm.

As always in such circumstances, the time seemed to pass inordinately slowly, but in reality she had not been there more than a quarter of an hour before she observed the figure of a man emerge from some trees, a few hundred yards distant, and come towards her, and despite the fact that he was wearing a raincoat, with the collar turned up to his ears, and a tweed cap pulled well down over his head, she had no difficulty in recognizing in the approaching figure her fellow-traveller of the journey to Monkshaven.

Evidently he had not seen her, for she could hear him whistling softly to himself as he approached, while with the fingers of one hand he drummed on his chest as though beating out the rhythm of the melody he was whistling--a wild, passionate refrain from Wieniawski's exquisite **Legende**. It sounded curiously in harmony with the tempest that raged about him.

For himself, he appeared to regard the storm with indifference--almost to welcome it, for more than once Sara saw him raise his head as though he were glad to feel the wind and rain beating against his face.

She drew back a little into the shadows of the summer-house, hoping he might turn aside without observing her, since, from all accounts, Garth Trent was hardly the type of man to welcome a trespasser upon his property.

But he came straight on towards her, and an instant later she knew that her presence was discovered, for he stopped abruptly and peered through the driving rain in the direction of the summer-house. Then, quickening his steps, he rapidly covered the intervening space and halted on the threshold of the shelter.

"What the devil----" he began, then paused and stared down at her with an odd glint of amusement in his eyes. "So it's you, is it?" he said at last, with a short laugh.

Once again Sara was conscious of the extraordinary intensity of his regard, and now, as a sudden ragged gleam of sunlight pierced the clouds, falling athwart his face, she realized what it was that induced it. In both eyes the clear hazel of the iris was broken by a tiny, irregularly shaped patch of vivid blue, close to the pupil, and its effect was to give that curious depth and intentness of expression which Molly had tried to describe when she had said that Garth Trent's were the kind of eyes which "make you jump if he looked at you suddenly."

Sara almost jumped now; then, supported by her indignant recollection of the man's churlishness on a former occasion, she bowed silently.

He continued to regard her with that lurking suggestion of amusement at the back of his eyes, and she was annoyed to feel herself flushing uncomfortably beneath his scrutiny. At last he spoke again.

"You seem to have a faculty for intrusion," he remarked drily.

Sara's eyes flashed.

"And you, a fancy for solitude," she retorted.

"Exactly." He bowed ironically. "Perhaps you would oblige me by considering it?" And he drew politely aside as though to let her pass out in front of him.

Sara cast a dismayed glance at the rain, which was still descending in torrents. Then she turned to him indignantly.

"Do you mean that you're going to insist on my starting out in this storm?" she demanded.

"Don't you know that you've no right to be here at all--that you're trespassing?" he parried coolly.

"Of course I know it! But I didn't expect that any one in the world would object to my trespassing in the circumstances!"

"You must not judge me by other people," he replied composedly. "I am not--like them."

"You're not, indeed," agreed Sara warmly.

"And your tone implies 'thanks be,'" he supplemented with a faint smile. "Oh, well," he went on ungraciously, "stay if you like--so long as you don't expect me to stay with you."

Sara hastily disclaimed any such desire, and, lifting his cap, he turned and strode away into the rain.

Another ten minutes crawled by, and still the rain came down as persistently as though it intended never to cease again. Sara fidgeted, and walked across impatiently to the open front of the summer-house, staring up moodily at the heavy clouds. They showed no signs of breaking, and she was just about to resume her weary waiting on the seat within the shelter, when quick steps sounded to her left, and Garth Trent reappeared, carrying an umbrella and with a man's overcoat thrown over his arm.

"It's going to rain for a good two hours yet," he said abruptly. "You'd better come up to the house."

Sara gazed at him in silent amazement; the invitation was so totally unexpected that for the moment she had no answer ready.

"Unless," he added sneeringly, misinterpreting her silence, "you're afraid of the proprieties?"

"I'm far more afraid of taking cold," she replied promptly, preparing to evacuate the summer-house.

"Here, put this on," he said gruffly, holding out the coat he had brought with him. "There's no object in getting any wetter than you must."

He helped her into the coat, buttoning it carefully under her chin, his dexterous movements and quiet solicitude contrasting curiously with the detachment of his manner whilst performing these small services. He was so altogether business-like and unconcerned that Sara felt not unlike a child being dressed by a conscientious but entirely disinterested nurse. When he had fastened the last button of the long coat, which came down to her heels, he unfurled the umbrella and held it over her.

"Keep close to me, please," he said briefly, nor did he volunteer any further remark until they had accomplished the journey to the house, and were standing together in the old-fashioned hall which evidently served him as a living room.

Here Trent relieved her of the coat, and while she stood warming her feet at the huge log-fire, blazing half-way up the chimney, he rang for his servant and issued orders for tea to be brought, as composedly as though visitors of the feminine persuasion were a matter of everyday occurrence.

Sara, catching a glimpse of Judson's almost petrified face of astonishment as he retreated to carry out his master's instructions, and with a vivid recollection of her last encounter with him, almost laughed out loud.

"Please sit down," said Trent. "And"--with a glance towards her feet--"you had better take off those wet shoes."

There was something in his curt manner of giving orders--rather as though he were a drill-sergeant, Sara reflected--that aroused her to opposition. She held out her feet towards the blaze of the fire.

"No, thank you," she replied airily. "They'll dry like this."

As she spoke, she glanced up and encountered a sudden flash in his eyes like the keen flicker of a sword-blade. Without vouchsafing any answer, he knelt down beside her and began to unlace her shoes, finally drawing them off and laying them sole upwards, in front of the fire to dry. Then he passed his hand lightly over her stockinged feet.

"Wringing wet!" he remarked curtly. "Those silk absurdities must come off as well."

Sara sprang up.

"No!" she said firmly. "They shall not!"

He looked at her, again with that glint of mocking amusement with which he had first greeted her presence in his summer-house.

"You'd rather have a bad cold?" he suggested.

"Ever so much rather!" retorted Sara hardily.

He gave a short laugh, almost as though he could not help himself, and, with a shrug of his shoulders, turned and marched out of the room.

Left alone, Sara glanced about her in some surprise at the evidences of a cultivated taste and love of beauty which the room supplied. It was not quite the sort of abode she would have associated with the grim, misanthropic type of man she judged her host to be.

The old-fashioned note, struck by the huge oaken beams supporting the ceiling and by the open hearth, had been retained throughout, and every detail--the blue willow-pattern china on the old oak dresser, the dimly lustrous pewter perched upon the chimney-piece, the silver candle-sconces thrusting out curved, gleaming arms from the paneled walls--was exquisite of its kind. It reminded her of the old hall at Barrow, where she and Patrick had been wont to sit and yarn together on winter evenings.

The place had a well-tended air, too, and Sara, who waged daily war against the slovenly shabbiness prevalent at Sunnyside, was all at once sensible of how desperately she had missed the quiet perfection of the service at Barrow. The nostalgia for her old home--the unquenchable, homesick longing for the *place* that has held one's happiness--rushed over her in a overwhelming flood.

Wishing she had never come to this house, which had so stirred old memories, she got up restlessly, driven by a sudden impulse to escape, just as the door opened to re-admit Garth Trent.

He gave her a swift, searching glance.

"Sit down again," he commanded. "There"--gravely depositing a towel and a pair of men's woolen socks on the floor beside her--"dry your feet and put those socks on."

He moved quickly away towards the window and remained there, with his back turned studiously towards her, while she obeyed his instructions. When she had hung two very damp black silk stockings on the fire-dogs to dry, she flung a somewhat irritated glance at him over her shoulder.

"You can come back," she said in a small voice.

He came, and stood staring down at the two woolly socks protruding from beneath the short, tweed skirt. The suspicion of a smile curved his lips.

"They're several sizes too large," he observed. "Odd creatures you women are," he went on suddenly, after a brief silence. "You shy wildly at the idea of letting a man see the foot God gave you, but you've no scruples at all about letting any one see the selfishness that the devil's put into your hearts."

He spoke with a kind of savage contempt; it was as though the speech were tinged with some bitter personal memory.

Sara's eyes surveyed him calmly.

"I've no intention of making an exhibit of my heart," she observed mildly.

"It's wiser not, probably," he retorted disagreeably, and at that moment Judson came into the room and began to arrange the tea-table beside his master's chair.

"Put it over there," directed Trent sharply, indicating with a gesture that the table should be placed near his guest, and Judson, his face manifesting rather more surprise than is compatible with the wooden mask demanded of the well-trained servant, hastened to comply.

When he had readjusted the position of the tea-table, he moved quietly about the room, drawing the curtains and lighting the candles in their silver sconces, so that little pools of yellow light splashed down on to the smooth surface of the oak floor--waxed and polished till it gleamed like black ivory.

As he withdrew unobtrusively towards the door, Trent tossed him a further order.

"I shall want the car round in a couple of hours--at six," he said, and smiled straight into Sara's startled eyes.

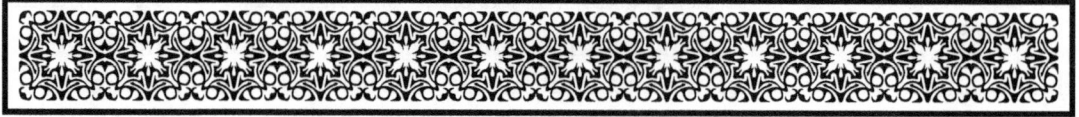

CHAPTER IX
THE HERMIT'S SHELL

Sara paused with the sugar-tongs poised above the Queen Anne bowl.

"Sugar?" she queried.

Trent regarded her seriously.

"One lump, please."

She handed him his cup and poured out another for herself. Then she said lightly:

"I heard you order your car. Is this quite a suitable afternoon for joy-riding?"

"More so than for walking," he retaliated. "I'm going to drive you home."

"At six o'clock?"

"At six o'clock."

"And suppose I wish to leave before then?"

He cast an expressive glance towards the windows, where the rain could be heard beating relentlessly against the panes.

"It's quite up to you . . . to walk home."

Sara made a small grimace of disgust.

"Otherwise," she said tentatively, "I am going to stay here, whether I will or no?"

He nodded.

"Yes. It's my birthday, and I'm proposing to make myself a present of an hour or two of your society," he replied composedly.

Sara regarded him with curiosity. He had been openly displeased to find her trespassing on his estate--which was only what current report would have led her to expect--yet now he was evincing a desire for her company, and, in addition, a very determined intention to secure it. The man was an enigma!

"I'm surprised," she said lightly. "I gathered from a recent remark of yours that you didn't think too highly of women."

"I don't," he replied with uncompromising directness.

"Then why--why----"

"Perhaps I have a fancy to drop back for a brief space into the life I have renounced," he suggested mockingly.

"Then you really are what they call you--a hermit?"

"I really am."

"And feminine society is taboo?"

"Entirely--as a rule." If, for an instant, the faintest of smiles modified the grim closing of his lips, Sara failed to notice it.

The cold detachment of his answer irritated her. It was as though he intended to remain, hermit-like, within his shell, and she had a suspicion that behind this barricade he was laughing at her for her ineffectual attempts to dig him out of it with a pin.

"I suppose some woman didn't fall into your arms just when you wanted her to?" she hazarded.

She had not calculated the result of this thrust. His eyes blazed for a moment. Then, a shade of contempt blending with the former cool insouciance of his tone, he said quietly:

"You don't expect an answer to that question, do you?"

The snub was unmistakable, and Sara's cheeks burned. She felt heartily ashamed of herself, and yet, incongruously, she was half inclined to lay the blame for her impertinent speech on his shoulders. He had almost challenged her to deal a blow that should crack that impervious shell of his.

She glanced across at him beneath her lashes, and in an instant all thought of personal dignity was wiped out by the look of profound pain that she surprised in his face. Her shrewd question, uttered almost unthinkingly in the cut-and-thrust of repartee, had got home somewhere on an old wound.

"Oh, I'm sorry!" she exclaimed contritely.

She could only assume that he had not heard her low-voiced apology, for, when he turned to her again, he addressed her exactly as though she had not spoken.

"Try some of these little hot cakes," he said, tendering a plateful. "They are quite one of Mrs. Judson's specialties."

With amazing swiftness he had reassumed his mask. The bright, hazel eyes were entirely free from any hint of pain, and his voice held nothing more than conventional politeness. Sara meekly accepted one of the cakes in question, and for a little while the conversation ran on stereotyped lines.

Presently, when tea was over, he offered her a cigarette.

"I have not forgotten your tastes, you see," he said, smiling.

"I do smoke," she admitted. "But"--the confession came with a rush, and she did not quite know what impelled her to make it--"I smoked--that day in the train--out of sheer defiance."

"I was sure of it," he responded in amused tones. "But now"--striking a match and holding it for her to light her cigarette--"you will smoke because you really like it, and because it would be a friendly action and condone the fact that you are being held a prisoner against your will."

Sara smiled.

"It is a very charming prison," she said, contemplating the harmony of the room with satisfied eyes.

"You like it?" he asked eagerly.

She looked at him in surprise. What could it matter to him whether she liked it or not?

"Why, of course, I like it," she replied. "Who wouldn't? You see," she added a little wistfully, "I have no home of my own now, so I have to enjoy other people's."

"I have no home, either," he said shortly.

"But--but this----"

"Is the house in which I live. One wants more than a few sticks of furniture to make a home."

Sara was struck by the intense bitterness in his tone. Truly this man, with his lightning changes from boorish incivility to whole-hearted hospitality, from apparently impenetrable reserve to an almost desperate outspokenness, was as incomprehensible as any sphinx.

She hastily steered the conversation towards a less dangerous channel, and gradually they drifted into the discussion of art and music; and Sara, not without some inward trepidation--remembering Molly's experience--touched on his own musicianship.

"It was surely you I herd?" she queried a trifle hesitatingly. "You were playing some Russian music that I knew. Your man ordered me off the premises"--smiling a little--"so I didn't hear as much as I should have liked."

"Is that a hint?" he asked whimsically.

"A broad one. Please take it."

He hesitated a moment. Then--

"Very well," he said abruptly.

He rose and led the way into an adjoining room.

Like the hall they had just quitted, it was pleasantly illumined by candles in silver sconces, and had evidently been arranged to serve exclusively as a music-room, for it contained practically no furniture beyond a couple of chairs, and a beautiful mahogany cabinet, of which the doors stood open, revealing sliding shelves crammed full of musical scores.

A grand piano was so placed that the light from either window or candles would fall comfortably upon the music-desk; and on a stool beside it rested a violin case.

Trent opened the case, and, lifting the violin from is cushiony bed of padded satin, fingered it caressingly.

"Can you read accompaniments?" he asked, flashing the question at her with his usual abruptness.

"Yes." Sara's answer came simply, minus the mock-modest tag: "A little," or "I'll do my best," which most people seem to think it incumbent on them to add, in the circumstances.

It is one of the mysteries of convention why, when you are perfectly aware that you can do a thing, and do it well, you are expected to depreciate your capability under penalty of being accounted overburdened with conceit should you fail to do so.

"Good." Trent pulled out an armful of music from the cabinet and looked through it rapidly.

"We'll have some of these." ("These" being several suites for violin and piano.)

Sara's lips twitched. He was testing her rather highly, since the pianoforte score of the suites in question was by no means easy. But, thanks to the wisdom of

Patrick Lovell, who had seen to it that she studied under one of the finest masters of the day, she was not a musician by temperament alone, but had also a surprisingly good technique.

At the close of the second suite, Trent turned to her enthusiastically, his face aglow. For the moment he was no longer the hermit, aloof and enigmatical, but an eager comrade, spontaneously appealing to a congenial spirit.

"That went splendidly, didn't it?" he exclaimed. "The pianoforte score is a pretty stiff one, but I was sure"--smilingly--"from the downright way you answered my question about accompaniments, that you'd prove equal to it."

Sara smiled back at him.

"I didn't think it necessary to make any conventional professions of modesty--to you," she said. "You don't--wrap things up much--yourself."

He leaned against the piano, looking down at her.

"No. Nothing I say can make things either better or worse for me, so I have at least gained freedom from the conventions. That is one of my few compensations."

"Compensations for what?" The question escaped her almost before she was aware, and she waited for the snub which she felt would inevitably follow her second indiscretion that afternoon.

But it did not come. Instead, he fenced adroitly.

"Compensation for the limitations of a hermit's life," he said lightly.

"The life is your own choice," she flashed back at him.

"Oh, no, we're not always given a choice, you know. This world isn't a kind of sublimated children's party."

She regarded him thoughtfully.

"I think," she said gravely, "we always get back out of life just what we put into it."

His mouth twisted ironically.

"That's a charming doctrine, but I'm afraid I can't subscribe to it. I put in--all my capital. And I've drawn a blank."

His tone implied a kind of strange, numb acceptance of an inimical destiny, and Sara was conscious of a rush of intense pity towards this man whose implacably cynical outlook manifested itself in almost every word he uttered. It was no mere pose on his part--of that she felt assured--but something ingrained, grafted on to his very nature by the happenings of life.

Rather girlishly she essayed to combat it.

"You're not at the end of life yet."

He smiled at her--a sudden, rare smile of extraordinary sweetness. Her intention was so unmistakable--so touchingly ingenious, as are all youth's attempts to heal a bitterness that lies beyond its ken.

"There are no more lucky dips left in life's tub for me, I'm afraid," he said gently.

Sara seized upon the opening afforded.

"Of course not--if you persist in keeping to the role of looker-on," she retorted.

He regarded her gravely.

"Unfortunately, I've no longer any right to dip my head into the tub. Even if I chanced to draw a prize--I should only have to put it back again."

The quiet irrevocableness of his answer shook her optimism.

"I--don't understand," she said hesitatingly.

"No?"--his tones hardened suddenly. "It's just as well you shouldn't, perhaps."

The abrupt alteration in his manner took her by surprise. All at once, he seemed to have retreated into his shell, to have become again the curt, ironic individual of their first meeting.

"I think," he went on, tranquilly ignoring the mixture of chagrin and amazement in her face, "I think I hear the car coming round. You had better put on your shoes and stockings again--they'll be dry now--and then we can start. It's no longer raining."

Sara felt as though she had been suddenly relegated to a position of utter unimportance. He was showing her that, as far as he was concerned, she was a person of not the slightest consequence, treating her like an inquisitive child. Their recent conversation, during which his mantle of reserve had slipped a little aside, the music they had shared, when for a brief time they had walked together in the pleasant paths of mutual understanding, all seemed to have receded an immense distance away. As she took her place in the car, she could almost have believed that the incidents of the afternoon were a dream, and nothing more.

Trent sat silently beside her, his attention apparently concentrated on the driving of the car. Once he asked her if she were warm enough, and, upon her replying in the affirmative, lapsed again into silence.

Gaining security from his abstraction, Sara ventured to steal a side-glance at his face. It was a curiously contradictory face, hard and bitter-looking, yet the reckless mouth curved sensitively at the corners, and the tolerant, humorous lines about the eyes seemed to combat the impression of almost brutal force conveyed by the frowning brows and square, dominant chin.

Always acutely sensible of temperament, Sara felt as though the man beside her might be capable of any extreme of action. Whatever decision he might adopt over any given matter, he would hold by it, come what may, and she was aware of an odd reflex consciousness of feminine inadequacy. To influence Garth Trent against his convictions would be like trying to deflect the course of a river by laying a straw across its track.

The primitive woman in her thrilled a little, responsively, and she wondered whether or no her sex had played much part in his life. He was a woman-hater--so Molly had told her--yet Sara could imagine him in a very different role. Of one thing she was sure--that the woman who was loved by Garth Trent would anchor in no placid back-water. Life, for her, would hold something breathless, vital, ex-ultant . . .

"Well, have you decided yet?"

The ironical voice broke sharply into the midst of her fugitive thoughts, and Sara jumped violently, flushing scarlet as she found Trent's eyes surveying her with a quietly quizzical expression.

"Decided what?" she asked defensively.

"Where to place me--whether among the sheep or the goats. You were dissect-ing my character, weren't you?"

He waited for an answer, but Sara maintained an embarrassed silence. He had divined the subject of her thoughts too nearly.

He laughed.

"The decision has gone against me, I see. Well, I'm not surprised. I've certainly treated you with a rather rough-and-ready kind of courtesy. You must try to pardon me. A hermit gets little practice at entertaining angels unawares."

Sara, recovering her composure, regarded him placidly.

"You might find many opportunities for practice in Monkshaven," she suggested.

"In Monkshaven? Are you trying to suggest that I should ingratiate myself with the leading lights of local society?"

She nodded.

"Why not?"

He laughed as though genuinely amused.

"Perhaps you've not been here long enough yet to discover that the amiable inhabitants of Monkshaven look upon me as a sort of cross between a madman and a criminal who has eluded justice."

"Whose fault is that?"

"Oh, mine, I suppose"--quickly. "But it doesn't matter--since I regard them as a set of harmless, conventional fools. No, thank you, I've no intention of making friends with the people of Monkshaven."

"They're not all conventional. Some of them are rather interesting--Mrs. Maynard, for instance, and the Herricks."

He gave her a keen glance.

"Do you know the Herricks?"

"Yes. Why don't you go to see them sometimes? Miles--"

"Oh, Miles Herrick's all right. I know that," he interrupted.

"It's very bad for you to cut yourself off from the rest of the world, as you do," persisted Sara sagely.

He was silent for a while, his eyes intent on the strip of road that stretched in front of him, and when he spoke again it was to draw her attention to the effect of the cloud shadows moving across the sea, exactly as though nothing of greater interest had been under discussion.

She began to recognize as a trick of his this abrupt method of terminating a conversation that for some reason did not please him. It was as conclusive as when the man at the other end of the 'phone suddenly "rings off" without any preliminary warning.

By this time they had reached the steep hill that approached directly to the Selwyns' house, and a couple of minutes later, Trent brought the car to a standstill at the gate.

"You have nothing to thank me for," he said, curtly dismissing her expression of thanks as they stood together on the path. "It is I who should be grateful to you. My opportunities of social intercourse"--drily--"are somewhat limited."

"Extend them, then, as I advised," retorted Sara.

"Do you wish me to?" he asked swiftly, and his intent eyes sought her face with a sudden hawk-like glance.

Her own eyes fell. She was conscious, all at once, of an inexplicable agitation, a tremulous confusion that made it seem a physical impossibility to reply.

But he still waited for his answer, and, at last, with an effort she mastered the nervousness that had seized her.

"I--I--yes, I do wish it," she said faintly.

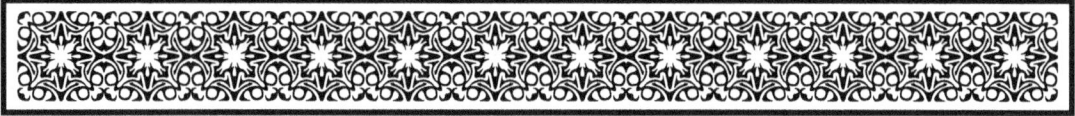

CHAPTER X
A MEETING AT ROSE COTTAGE

It had not taken Sara very long to cut a niche for herself in the household at Sunnyside. In a dwelling where the master of the house was away the greater part of the day, the mistress a chronic invalid, and the daughter a beautiful young thing whose mind was intent upon "colour" and "atmosphere," and altogether hazy concerning the practical necessities of housekeeping, the advent of any one possessing even half Sara's intelligent efficiency would have been provocative of many reforms.

Dick Selwyn, pushed to the uttermost limits of his strength by the demands of his wide practice and by the nervous strain of combating his wife's incessant fretfulness, quickly learned to turn to Sara for that sympathetic understanding which had hitherto been denied him in his home-life.

He had, of course, never again discussed with her his wife's incurable self-absorption, as on the day of her arrival, when the painful scene created by Mrs. Selwyn had practically forced him into some sort of explanation, but Sara's quick grasp of the situation had infinitely simplified matters, and by devoting a considerable amount of her own time to the entertainment of the captious invalid, and thus keeping her in a good humour, she contrived to save Selwyn many a bad half-hour of recrimination and complaint.

Sara was essentially a good "comrade," as Patrick Lovell had recognized in the old days at Barrow Court, and instinctively Selwyn came to share with her the pin-prick worries that dog a man's footsteps in this vale of woe, learning to laugh at them; and even his apprehensions concerning Molly's ultimate development and welfare were lessened by the knowledge that Sara was at hand.

Molly herself seemed to float through life like a big, beautiful moth, sailing serenely along, and now and then blundering into things, but never learning by experience the dangers of such blunders. One day, in the course of her inconsequent path through life, she would probably flutter too near the attractive blaze of some perilous fire, just as a moth flies against the flame of a candle and singes its frail, soft wings in the process.

It was of this that Sara was inwardly afraid, realizing, perhaps more clearly than the girl's overworked and sometimes absent-minded father, the risks attaching to her temperament.

Of late, Molly had manifested a certain moodiness and irritability very unlike her usual facile sweetness of disposition, and Sara was somewhat nonplussed to account for it. Finally, she approached the matter by way of a direct inquiry.

"What's wrong, Molly?"

Molly was hunched up in the biggest and shabbiest armchair by the fire, smoking innumerable cigarettes and flinging them away half-finished. At Sara's question, she looked up with a shade of defiance in her eyes.

"Why should anything be wrong?" she countered, obviously on the defensive.

"I don't know, I'm sure," responded Sara good-humouredly. "But I'm pretty certain there is something. Come, out with it, you great baby!"

Molly sighed, smoked furiously for a moment, and then tossed her cigarette into the fire.

"Well, yes," she admitted at last. "There is--something wrong." She rose and stood looking across at Sara like a big, perplexed child. "I--I owe some money."

Sara was conscious of a distinct shock.

"How much?" she asked sharply.

"It's--it's rather a lot--twenty pounds!"

"Twenty pounds!" This was certainly a large sum for Molly--whose annual dress allowance totaled very little more--to be in debt. "What on earth have you been up to? Buying a new trousseau? Where do you owe it--Carr & Bishop's?"-- mentioning the principal draper's shop in Oldhampton.

"No. I--don't owe it to a shop at all. It's--it's a bridge debt!" The confession came out rather hurriedly.

Sara's face grew grave.

"But, Molly, you little fool, you've no business to be playing bridge. Where have you been playing?"

"Oh, we play sometimes at the studios--when the light's too bad to go on painting, you know"--airily.

"You mean," said Sara, "the artists' club people play?"

"Yes."

Sara frowned. She knew that Molly was one of the youngest members of this club of rather irresponsible and happy-go-lucky folk, and privately considered that Selwyn had made a great mistake in ever allowing her to join it. It embodied, as she had discovered by inquiry, some of the most rapid elements of Oldhampton's society, and was, moreover, open to receive as temporary members artists who come from other parts of the country to paint in the neighbourhood. More than one well-known name had figured in the temporary membership list, and, in addition, the name of certain **dilettanti** to whom the freedom from convention of the artistic life signified far more that art itself.

"I don't understand," said Sara slowly, "how they let you go on playing until you owed twenty pounds. Don't you square up at the end of the afternoon's play?"

"Yes. But I'd--I'd been losing badly, and--and some one lent me the money."

Molly flushed a bewitching rose-colour and appealed with big, pathetic eyes. It was difficult to be righteously wroth with her, but Sara steeled her heart.

"You'd no right to borrow," she said shortly.

"No. I know I hadn't. But, don't you see, I thought I should be sure to win it all back? I couldn't ask Dad for it. Every penny he can spare goes on something that mother can't possibly do without," added the girl with unwonted bitterness.

The latter fact was incontrovertible, and Sara remained silent. In her own mind she regarded Mrs. Selwyn as a species of vampire, sucking out all that was good, and sweet, and wholesome from the lives of those about her--even that of her own daughter. Did the woman realize, she wondered, that instead of being the help all mothers were sent into the world to be, she was nothing but a hindrance and a stumbling-block?

"I don't know what to do, I simply don't." Molly's humble, dejected tones broke through the current of Sara's thoughts. "You see, the worst of it is"--she blushed even more bewitchingly than before--"that I owe it to a **man**. It's detestable owing money to a man!"--with suppressed irritation.

Two fine lines drew themselves between Sara's level brows. This was worse than she had imagined.

"Who is it?" she asked, at last, quietly.

"Lester Kent."

"And who--or what--is Lester Kent?"

"He's--he's an artist--by choice. I mean," stumbled Molly, "that he's quite well off--he only paints for pleasure. He often runs down from town for a month or two at a time and takes out a temporary membership for our club."

"And he has lent you this money?"

"Yes"--rather shamefacedly.

"Well, he must be paid back at once. At once, do you understand? I will give you the twenty pounds--you're not to bother your father about it."

"Oh, Sara! You are a blessed duck!"

In an instant Molly's cares had slipped from her shoulders, and she beamed across at her deliverer with the most disarming gratitude.

"Wait a moment," continued Sara firmly. "You must never borrow from Mr. Kent--or any one else--again."

"Oh, I won't! Indeed, I won't!" Molly was fervent in her assurances. "I've been wretched over this. Although"--brightening--"Lester Kent was really most awfully nice about it. He said it didn't matter one bit."

"Did he indeed?" Sara spoke rather grimly. "And how old is this Lester Kent?"

"How old? Oh"--vaguely--"thirty-five--forty, perhaps. I really don't know. Somehow he's not the sort of person whose age one thinks about."

"Anyway, he's old enough to know better than to be lending you money to play bridge with," commented Sara. "I wish you'd give up playing, Molly."

"Oh, I couldn't!" coaxingly. "We play for very small stakes--as a rule. But it *is* amusing, Sara. And, you know this place is as dull as ditchwater unless one does *something*. But I won't get into debt again--I really won't."

Molly had all the caressing charm of a nice kitten, and now that the pressing matter of her indebtedness to Lester Kent was settled, she relapsed into her usual tranquil, happy-go-lucky self. She rubbed her cheek confidingly against Sara's.

"You are a pet angel, Sara, my own," she said. "I'm so glad you adopted us. Now I can go to the Herricks' tea-party this afternoon without having that twenty pounds nagging at the back of my mind all the time. I suppose"--glancing at the clock--"it's time we put on our glad rags. The Lavender Lady said she expected us at four."

Half-an-hour later, Molly reappeared, looking quite impossibly lovely in a frock of the cheapest kind of material, "run up" by the local dressmaker, and very evidently with no other thought "at the back of her mind" than of the afternoon's entertainment.

The tea-party was a small one, commensurate with the size of the rooms at Rose Cottage, and included only Sara and Molly, Mrs. Maynard, and, to Sara's surprise, Garth Trent.

As she entered the room, he turned quietly from the window where he had been standing looking out at the Herricks' charming garden.

"Mr. Trent"--Miss Lavinia fluttered forward--"let me introduce you to Miss Tennant."

The Lavender Lady's pretty, faded blue eyes beamed benevolently on him. She was so **very** glad that "that poor, lonely fellow at Far End" had at last been induced to desert the solitary fastnesses of Monk's Cliff, but as she was simply terrified at the prospect of entertaining him herself--and Audrey Maynard seemed already fully occupied, chatting with Miles--she was only too thankful to turn him across to Sara's competent hands.

"We've met before, Miss Lavinia," said Trent, and over her head his hazel eyes met Sara's with a gamin amusement dancing in them. "Miss Tennant kindly called on me at Far End."

"Oh, I didn't know." Little Miss Lavinia gazed in a puzzled fashion from one to the other of her guests. "Sara, my dear, you never told me that you and Dr. Selwyn had called on Mr. Trent."

Sara laughed outright.

"Dear Lavender Lady--we didn't. Neither of us would have dared to insult Mr. Trent by doing anything so conventional." The black eyes flashed back defiance at the hazel ones. "I got caught in a storm on the Monk's Cliff, and Mr. Trent--much against his will, I'm certain"--maliciously--"offered me shelter."

"Now that was kind of him. I'm sure Sara must have been most grateful to you." And the kind old face smiled up into Trent's dark, bitter one so simply and sincerely that it seemed as though, for the moment, some of the bitterness melted away. Not even so confirmed a misanthrope as the hermit of Far End could have entirely resisted the Lavender Lady, with her serene aroma of an old-world courtesy and grace long since departed from these hurrying twentieth-century days.

She moved away to the tea-table, leaving Trent and Sara standing together in the bay of the window.

"So you are overcoming your distaste for visiting," said Sara a little nervously. "I didn't expect to meet you here."

His glance held hers.

"You wished it," he answered gravely.

A sudden colour flamed up into the warm pallor of her skin.

"Are you suggesting I invited you to meet me here?" she responded, willfully misinterpreting him. She shook her read regretfully. "You must have misunderstood me. I should never have imposed such a strain on your politeness."

His eyes glinted.

"Do you know," he said quietly, "that I should very much like to shake you?"

"I'm glad," she answered heartily. "It's a devastating feeling! You made me feel just the same the day I travelled with you. So now we're quits."

"Won't you--please--try to forget that day in the train?" he said quickly. "I behaved like a bore. I'm afraid I've no real excuse to offer, except that I'd been reminded of something that happened long ago--and I wanted to be alone."

"To enjoy the memory in solitude?" hazarded Sara flippantly. She was still nervous and talking rather at random, scarcely heeding what she said.

A look of bitter irony crossed his face.

"Hardly that," he said shortly, and Sara knew that somehow she had again inadvertently laid her hand upon an old hurt. She spoke with a sudden change of voice.

"Then, as the train doesn't hold pleasant memories for either of us, let's forget it," she suggested gently.

"Do you know what that implies?" he asked. "It implies that you are willing to be friends. Do you mean that?"--incisively.

She nodded silently, not trusting herself to speak.

"Thank you," he said curtly, and then Audrey Maynard's gay voice broke across the tension of the moment.

"Mr. Trent, I simply cannot allow Sara to monopolize you any longer. Now that we **have** succeeded in dragging the hermit out of his shell, we all want a share of his society, please."

Trent turned instantly, and Sara slipped across the room and took the place Audrey had vacated by Miles's couch. He greeted her coming with a smile, but there were shadows of fatigue beneath his eyes, and his lips were rather white and drawn-looking.

"This is a lazy way to receive visitors, isn't it?" he said apologetically. "But my game leg's given out to-day, so you must forgive me."

Sara's glance swept his face with quick sympathy.

"You oughtn't to be at the 'party' at all," she said. "You look far too tired to be bothered with a parcel of chattering women."

He smiled.

"Do you know," he whispered humorously, "that, although you're quite the four nicest women I know, the shameful truth is that I'm really here on behalf of the one man! I met him yesterday in the town and booked him for this afternoon, and, having at last dislodged him from his lone pinnacle, I hadn't the heart to leave him unsupported."

"No. I'm glad you dug him out, Miles. It was clever of you."

"It will give Monkshaven something to talk about, anyway"--whimsically.

"I suppose"--the toe of Sara's narrow foot was busily tracing a pattern on the carpet--"I suppose you don't know why he shuts himself up like that at Far End?"

"No, I don't," he answered. "But I'd wager it's for some better reason than people give him credit for. Or it may be merely a preference for his own society. Anyway, it is no business of ours." Then, swiftly softening the suggestion of reproof contained in his last sentence, he added: "Don't encourage me to gossip, Sara. When a man's tied by the leg, as I am, it's all he can do to curb a tendency towards tattling village scandal like some garrulous old woman."

It was evident that the presence of visitors was inflicting a considerable strain on Herrick's endurance, and, as though by common consent, the little party broke up shortly after tea.

Molly expressed her intention of accompanying Mrs. Maynard back to Greenacres--the beautiful house which the latter had had built to her own design, over-looking the bay--in order to inspect the pretty widow's recent purchase of a new motor-car.

Trent turned to Sara with a smile.

"Then it devolves on me to see you safely home, Miss Tennant, may I?"

She nodded permission, and they set off through the high-hedged lane, Sara hurrying along at top speed.

For a few minutes Trent strode beside her in silence. Then:

"Are you catching a train?" he inquired mildly. "Or is it only that you want to be rid of my company in the shortest possible time?"

She coloured, moderating her pace with an effort. Once again the odd nervousness engendered by his presence had descended on her. It was as though something in the man's dominating personality strung all her nerves to a high tension of consciousness, and she felt herself overwhelmingly sensible of his proximity.

He smiled down at her.

"Then--if you're not in any hurry to get home--will you let me take you round by Crabtree Moor? It's part of a small farm of mine, and I want a word with my tenant."

Sara acquiesced, and, Trent, having speedily transacted the little matter of business with his tenant, they made their way across a stretch of wild moorland which intersected the cultivated fields lying on either hand.

In the dusk of the evening, with the wan light of the early moon deepening the shadows and transforming the clumps of furze into strange, unrecognizable shapes of darkness, it was an eerie enough place. Sara shivered a little, instinctively moving closer to her companion. And then, as they rounded a furze-crowned hummock, out of the hazy twilight, loping along on swift, padding feet, emerged the figure of a man.

With a muttered curse he swerved aside, but Trent's arm shot out, and, catching him by the shoulder, he swung him round so that he faced them.

"Leggo!" he muttered, twisting in Trent's iron grasp. "Leggo, can't you?"

"I can, but I'm not going to," said Trent coolly. "At least, not till you've explained your presence here. This is private property. What are you doing on it?"

"I'm doing no harm," growled the man sullenly.

"No?" Trent passed his free hand swiftly down the fellow's body, feeling the bulge of his coat. "Then what's the meaning of those rabbits sticking out under your coat? Now, look here, my man, I know you. You're Jim Brady, and it's not the first, nor the second, time I've caught you poaching on my land. But it's the last. Understand that? This time the Bench shall deal with you."

The man was silent for a moment. Then suddenly he burst out:

"Look here, sir, pass it over this time. My missus is ill. She's mortal bad, God's truth she is, and haven't eaten nothing this three days past. An' I thought mebbe a bit o' stewed rabbit 'ud tempt 'er."

"Pshaw!" Trent was beginning contemptuously, when Sara leaned forward, peering into the poacher's face.

"Why," she exclaimed. "It's Brady--Black Brady from Fallowdene."

Ne'er-do-well as he was, the mere fact that he came from Fallowdene warmed her heart towards him.

"Yes, miss, that's so," he answered readily. "And you're the young lady what used to live at Barrow Court."

"Do you know this man?" Trent asked her.

"'Bout as well as you do, sir," volunteered Brady with an impudent grin. "Catched me poachin' one morning. Fired me gun at 'er, too, I did, to frighten 'er," he continued reminiscently. "And she never blinked. You're a good-plucked 'un, miss,"--with frank admiration.

Sara looked at the man doubtfully.

"I didn't know you lived here," she said.

"It's my native village, miss, Monks'aven is. But I didn't think 'twas too 'healthy for me down here, back along"--grinning--"so I shifted to Fallowdene, where me grandmother lives. I came back here to marry Bessie Windrake' she've stuck to me like a straight 'un. But I didn't mean to get collared poachin' again. Me and Bess was goin' to live respectable. 'Twas her bein' ill and me out of work w'at did it."

"Let him go," said Sara, appealing to Trent. But he shook his head.

"I can't do that," he answered with decision.

"Not 'im, miss, 'e won't," broke in Brady. "'E's not the soft-'earted kind, isn't Mr. Trent."

Trent's brows drew together ominously.

"You won't mend matters by impudence, Brady," he said sharply. "Get along now"--releasing his hold of the man's arm--"but you'll hear of this again."

Brady shot away into the darkness like an arrow, probably chortling to himself that his captor had omitted to relieve him of the brace of rabbits he had poached; and Sara, turning again to Trent, renewed her plea for clemency.

But Trent remained adamant.

"Why shouldn't he stand his punishment like any other man?" he said.

"Well, if it's true that his wife is ill, and that he has been out of work--"

"Are you offering those facts as an excuse for dishonesty?" asked Trent drily.

Sara smiled.

"Yes, I believe I am," she acknowledged.

He shrugged his shoulders.

"Like nine-tenths of your sex, you are fiercely Tory in theory and a rank socialist in practice," he grumbled.

"Well, I'm not sure that that isn't a very good working basis to go on," she retorted.

As they stood in the porch at Sunnyside, she made yet one more effort to smooth matters over for the evil-doer, but Trent's face still showed unrelenting in the light that streamed out through the open doorway.

"Ask me something else," he said. "I would do anything to please you, Sara, except"--with a sudden tense decision--"except interfere with the course of justice. Let every man pay the penalty for his own sin."

"That's a hard creed," objected Sara.

"Hard?" He shrugged his shoulders. "Perhaps it is. But"--grimly--"it's the only creed I believe in. Good-night"--he held out his hand abruptly. "I'm sorry I can't do as you ask about Jim Brady."

Before Sara could reply, he was striding away down the path, and a minute later the darkness had hidden him from view.

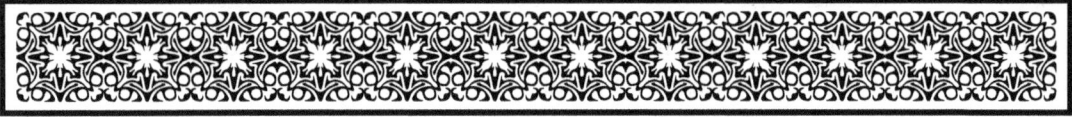

CHAPTER XI
TWO ON AN ISLAND

Sara's conviction that Garth Trent would not be easily turned from any decision that he might take had been confirmed very emphatically over the matter of Black Brady.

Notwithstanding the fact that the man's story of his wife's illness proved to be perfectly genuine, Trent persisted that he must take his punishment, and all that Sara could do by way of mitigation was to promise Brady that she would pay the amount of any fine which might be imposed.

Brady, however, was not optimistic.

"There'll be no opshun of a fine, miss," he told her. "I've a-been up before the gen'lemen too many times"--grinning. "But if so be you'd give an eye to Bessie here, whiles I'm in quod, I'd take it very kind of you."

His forecast summed up the situation with lamentable accuracy. No option of a fine was given, and during the brief space that the prison doors closed upon him, Sara saw to the welfare of his invalid wife, thereby winning the undying devotion of Black Brady's curiously composite soul.

When he again found himself at liberty, she induced the frankly unwilling proprietor of the Cliff Hotel--the only hotel of any pretension to which Monkshaven could lay claim--to take him into his employment as an odd-job man. How she accomplished this feat it is impossible to say, but the fact remains that she did accomplish it, and perhaps Jane Crab delved to the root of the matter in the terse comment which the circumstances elicited from her: "Miss Tennant has a way with her that 'ud make they stone sphinxes gallop round the desert if so be she'd a mind they should."

Apparently, however, the sphinx of Far End was compounded of even more adamantine substance than his feminine prototype, for he exhibited a mulish aversion to budging an inch--much less galloping--in the direction Sara had indicated as desirable.

The two quarreled vehemently over the matter, and a glacial atmosphere of hostility prevailed between them during the period of Black Brady's incarceration.

Garth, undeniably the victor, was the first to open peace negotiations, and a few days subsequent to Brady's release from prison, he waylaid Sara in the town.

She was preoccupied with numerous small, unnecessary commissions to be executed for Mrs. Selwyn at half-a-dozen different shops, and she would have passed him by with a frosty little bow had he not halted in front of her and deliberately held out his hand.

"Good-morning!" he said, blithely disregarding the coolness of his reception. "Am I still in disgrace? Brady's been restored to the bosom of his family for at least five days now, you know."

Overhead, the sun was shining gloriously in an azure sky flecked with little bunchy white clouds like floating pieces of cotton-wool, while an April breeze, fragrant of budding leaf and blossom, rollicked up the street. It seemed almost as though the frolicsome atmosphere of spring had permeated even the shell of the hermit and got into his system, for there was something incorrigibly boyish and youthful about him this morning. His cheerful smile was infectious.

"Can't I be restored, too?" he asked

"Restored to what?" asked Sara, trying to resist the contagion of his good humour.

"Oh, well"--a faint shadow dimmed the sparkle in his eyes--"to the same old place I held before our squabble over Brady--just friends, Sara."

For a moment she hesitated. He had pitted his will against hers and won, hands down, and she felt distinctly resentful. But she knew that in a strange, unforeseen way their quarrel had hurt her inexplicably. She had hated meeting the cool, aloof expression of his eyes, and now, urged by some emotion of which she was, as yet, only dimly conscious, she capitulated.

"That's good," he said contentedly. "And you might just as well give in now as later," he added, smiling.

"All the same," she protested, "you're a bully."

"I know I am--I glory in it! But now, just to show that you really do mean to be friends again, will you let me row you across to Devil's Hood Island this afternoon? You told me once that you wanted to go there."

Sara considered the proposition for a moment, then nodded consent.

"Yes, I'll come," she said, "I should like to."

Devil's Hood Island was a chip off the mainland which had managed to keep its head above water when the gradually encroaching sea had stolen yet another mile from the coast. Sandy dunes, patched here and there with clumps of coarse, straggling rushes, sloped upward from the rock-strewn shore to a big crag that crowned its further side--a curious natural formation which had given the island its name.

It was shaped like a great overhanging hood, out of which, crudely suggested by the configuration of the rock, peered a diabolical face, weather-worn to the smoothness of polished marble.

April was still doing her best to please, with blue skies and soft fragrant airs, when Garth gave a final push-off to the *Betsy Anne*, and bent to his oars as she skimmed out over the top of the waves with her nose towards Devil's Hood Island.

Sara, comfortably ensconced amid a nest of cushions in the stern of the boat, pointed to a square-shaped basket of quite considerable dimensions, tucked away beneath one of the seats.

"What's that?" she asked curiously.

Trent's eyes followed the direction of her glance.

"That? Oh, that's our tea. You didn't imagine I was going to starve you, did you? I think we shall find that Mrs. Judson has provided all we want."

Sara laughed across at him.

"What a thoughtful man you are!" she said gaily. "Fancy a hermit remembering a woman's crucial need of tea."

"Don't credit me with too much self-effacement!" he grinned. "I enjoyed the last occasion when you were my guest, so I'm repeating the prescription."

"Still, even deducting for the selfish motive, you're progressing," she answered. "I see you developing into quite an ornament to society in course of time."

"God forbid!" he ejaculated piously.

Sara looked entertained.

"Apparently your ambitions don't lie in that direction?" she rallied him.

"There is no question of such a catastrophe occurring. I've told you that society--as such--and I have finished with each other."

His face clouded over, and for a while he sculled in silence, driving the **Betsy Anne** through the blue water with strong, steady strokes.

Sara was vividly conscious of the suggestion of supple strength conveyed by the rippling play of muscle beneath the white skin of his arms, bared to the elbow, and by the pliant swing of his body to each sure, rhythmical stroke.

She recollected that one of her earliest impressions concerning him had been of the sheer force of the man--the lithe, flexible strength like that of tempered steel--and she wondered whether this were entirely due to his magnificent physique or owed its impulse, in part, to some mental quality in him. Her eyes travelled reflectively to the lean, square-jawed face, with its sensitive, bitter-looking mouth and its fine modeling of brow and temple, as though seeking there the answer to her questionings, and with a sudden, intuitive instinct of reliance, she felt that behind all his cynicism and surface hardness, there lay a quiet, sure strength of soul that would not fail whoever trusted it.

Yet he always spoke as though in some way his life had been a failure--as though he had met, and been defeated, by a shrewd blow of fate.

Sara found it difficult to associate the words failure and defeat with her knowledge of his dominating personality and force of will, and the natural curiosity which had been aroused in her mind by his strange mode of life, with its deliberate isolation, and by the aroma of mystery which seemed to cling about him, deepened.

Her brows drew together in a puzzled frown, as she inwardly sought for some explanation of the many inconsistencies she had encountered even in the short time that she had known him.

His abrupt alterations from reticence to unreserved; his avowed dislike of women and the contradictory enjoyment which he seemed to find in her society; his love of music and of beautiful surroundings--alike indicative of a cultivated appreciation and experience of the good things of this world--and the solitary, hermit-like existence which he yet chose to lead--all these incongruities of temperament and habit wove themselves into an enigma which she found impossible to solve.

"Here we are!"

Garth's voice recalled her abruptly from her musings to find that the **Betsy**

Anne was swaying gently alongside a little wooden landing-stage.

"But how civilized!" she exclaimed. "One does not expect to find a jetty on a desert-island."

Trent laughed grimly.

"Devil's Hood is far from being a desert island in the summer, when the tourists come this way. They swarm over it."

Whilst he was speaking, he had made fast the painter, and he now stepped out on to the landing-stage. Sara prepared to follow him. For a moment she stood poised with one foot on the gunwale of the boat, then, as an incoming wave drove the little skiff suddenly against the wooden supports of the jetty, she staggered, lost her balance, and toppled helplessly backward.

But even as she fell, Garth's arms closed round her like steel bars, and she felt herself lifted clean up from the rocking boat on to the landing-stage. For an instant she knew that she rested a dead weight against his breast; then he placed her very gently on her feet.

"All right?" he queried, steadying her with his hand beneath her arm. "That was a near shave."

His queer hazel eyes were curiously bright, and Sara, meeting their gaze, felt her face flame scarlet.

"Quite, thanks," she said a little breathlessly, adding: "You must be very strong."

She moved her arm as though trying to free it from his clasp, and he released it instantly. But his face was rather white as he knelt down to lift out the tea-basket, and he, too, was breathing quickly.

Somewhat silently they made their way up the sandy slope that stretched ahead of them, and presently, as they mounted the last rise, the malignant, distorted face beneath the Devil's Hood leaped into view, granite-grey and menacing against the young blue of the April sky.

"What a perfectly horrible head!" exclaimed Sara, gazing at it aghast. "It's like a nightmare of some kind."

"Yes, it's not pretty," admitted Garth. "The mouth has a sort of malevolent leer, hasn't it?"

"It has, indeed. One can hardly believe that it is just a natural formation."

"It's always a hotly debated point whether the devil and his hood are purely the work of nature or not. My own impression is that to a certain extent they are, but that someone--centuries ago--being struck by the resemblance of the rock to a human face, added a few touches to complete the picture."

"Well, whoever did it must have had a bizarre imagination to perpetuate such a thing."

"The handiwork--if handiwork it is--is attributed to Friar Anselmo--the Spanish monk who broke his vows and escaped to Monkshaven, you know."

Sara looked interested.

"No, I don't know," she said. "Tell me about him. He sounds quite exciting."

"You don't meant to say no one has enlightened you as to the gentleman whose exploit gave the town its name of Monkshaven?"

"No. I'm afraid my education as far as local history is concerned has been shamefully neglected. Do make good the deficiencies"--smiling.

Garth laughed a little.

"Very well, I will. I always have a kind of fellow-feeling for Friar Anselmo. But I propose we investigate the tea-basket first."

They established themselves beneath the shelter of a big boulder, Garth first spreading a rug which he had brought from the boat for Sara to sit on. Then he unstrapped the tea-basket, and it became evident either that Mrs. Judson had a genius for assembling together the most fascinating little cakes and savoury sandwiches, accompanied by fragrant tea, hot from a thermos flask, or else that she had acted under instructions from some one to whom the cult of afternoon tea as sublimated by Rumpelmayer was not an unknown quantity. Sara, sipping her tea luxuriously, decided in favour of the latter explanation.

"For a confirmed misogynist," she observed later on, when, the feast over, he was repacking the basket, "you have a very complete understanding of a woman's weakness for tea."

"It's a case of cause and effect. A misogynist"--caustically--"is the product of a very complete understanding of most feminine weaknesses."

Sara's slender figure tautened a little.

"Do you think," she said, speaking a little indignantly, "that it is quite nice of you to invite me out to a picnic and then to launch remarks of that description at my head?"

"No, I don't," he acknowledged bluntly. "It's making you pay some one else's bill." His lean brown hand closed suddenly over hers. "Forgive me, Sara!"

The abrupt intensity of his manner was out of all proportion to the merely surface friction of the moment; and Sara, sensing something deeper and of more significance behind it, hurriedly switched the conversation into a less personal channel.

"Very well," she said lightly, disengaging her hand. "I'll forgive you, and you shall tell me about Friar Anselmo." She lifted her eyes to the leering, sinister face that protruded from the Devil's Hood. "As, presumably, from his choice of a profession, he, too, had no love for women, you ought to enjoy telling his story," she added maliciously.

Garth's eyes twinkled.

"As a matter of fact, it was love o' women that was Anselmo's undoing," he said. "In spite of his vows, he fell in love--with a very beautiful Spanish lady, and to make matters worse, if that were possible, the lady was possessed of a typically jealous Spanish husband, who, on discovering how the land lay, killed his wife, and would have killed Anselmo as well, but that he escaped to England. The vessel on which he sailed was wrecked at the foot of what has been called, ever since, the Monk's Cliff; but Anselmo himself succeeded in swimming ashore, and spent the remainder of his life at Monkshaven, doing penance for the mistakes of his earlier days."

"He chose a charming place to repent in," said Sara, her eyes wandering to the distant bay, where the quaint little town straggled picturesquely up the hill that sloped away from the coast.

"Yes," responded Garth slowly, "it's not a bad place--to repent in. . . . It would be a better place still--to love and be happy in."

There was a brooding melancholy in his tones, and Sara, hearing it, spoke very gently.

"I hope you will find it--like that," she said.

"I?" He laughed hardly. "No! Those gifts of the gods are not for such as I. The husks are my portion. If it were not so"--his voice deepened to a sudden urgent note that moved her strangely--"if it were not so--"

As though in spite of himself, his arms moved gropingly towards her. Then, with a muttered exclamation, he turned away and sprang hastily to his feet.

"Let us go back," he said abruptly, and Sara, shaken by his vehemence, rose obediently, and they began to retrace their steps.

It had grown much colder. The sun hung low in the horizon, and the deceptive warmth of mid-afternoon had given place to the chill dampness in the atmosphere. Half unconsciously, feeling that the time must have slipped away more rapidly than she had suspected, Sara quickened her steps, Garth striding silently at her side. Presently the little wooden jetty came into view once more. It bore a curiously bare, deserted aspect, the waves riding and falling sluggishly on either side of its black, tarred planking, Sara stared at it incredulously, then an exclamation of sheer dismay burst from her lips.

"The boat! Look! It's gone!"

"*Gone?*" Garth's eyes sought the landing-stage, then swept the vista of grey-water ahead of them.

"*Damn!*" he ejaculated forcibly. "She's got adrift!"

A brown speck, bobbing maddeningly up and down in the distance and momentarily drifting further and further out to sea on the ebbing tide, was all that could be seen of the *Betsy Anne*.

An involuntary chuckle broke from Sara.

"Marooned!" she exclaimed. "How amusing!"

"Amusing?" Trent looked at her with a concerned expression. "It might be, if it were eleven o'clock in the morning. But it's the wrong end of the day. It will be dark before long." He paused, then asked swiftly: "Does any one at Sunnyside know where you are this afternoon?"

"No. The doctor and Molly were both out to lunch--and you know we only planned this trip this morning. I haven't seen them since. Why do you ask?"

"Because, if they know, they'd send over in search of us if we didn't turn up in the course of the next hour or so. But if they don't know where you are, we stand an excellent chance of spending the night here."

The gravity of what had first struck her as merely an amusing *contretemps* suddenly presented itself to Sara.

"Oh!--!" She drew her breath in sharply. "What--what on earth shall we do?"

"Do?" Garth spoke with grim force. "Why, you must be got off the island some-how. If not, you're fair game for every venomous tongue in the town."

"Would any one hear us from the shore if we shouted?" she suggested.

He shook his head.

"No. The sound would carry in the opposite direction to-day."

"Then what *can* we do?"

By this time the manifest anxiety in Trent's face was reflected in her own. The possibility that they might be compelled to spend the night on Devil's Hood Island was not one that could be contemplated with equanimity, for Sara had no illusions whatever as to the charitableness of the view the world at large would take of such an episode--however accidental its occurrence. Unfortunately, essential innocence is frequently but a poor tool wherewith to scotch a scandal.

"There is only one thing to be done," said Garth at last, after fruitlessly scanning the waters for any stray fishing-boat that might be passing. "I must swim across, and then row back and take you off."

"Swim across?" Sara regarded the distance between the island and the shore with consternation. "You couldn't possibly do it. It's too far."

"Just under a mile."

"But you would have the tide against you," she urged. The current off the coast ran with dangerous rapidity between the mainland and the island, and more than one strong swimmer, as Sara knew, had lost his life struggling against it.

She looked across to the further shore again, and all at once it seemed impossible to let Garth make the attempt.

"No! no! You can't go!" she exclaimed.

"You wouldn't be nervous at being alone here?" he asked doubtfully.

She stamped her foot.

"No! Of course not! But--oh! Don't you see? It's madness to think of swimming across with the tide against you! You could never do it. You might get cramp--Oh! Anything might happen! You shan't go!"

She caught his arm impetuously, her eyes dilating with the sudden terror that had laid hold of her. But he was obdurate.

"Look there," he said, pointing to a faint haze thickening the atmosphere. "Do you see the mist coming up? Very soon it will be all over us, like a blanket, and there'd be no possibility of swimming across at all. I must go at once."

"But that only adds to the danger," she argued desperately. "The fog may come down sooner than you expect, and then you'd lose your bearings altogether."

"I must risk that," he answered grimly. "Don't you realize that it's impossible--*impossible* for us to remain here?"

"No, I don't," she returned stubbornly. "It isn't worth such a frightful risk. Some one is sure to look for us eventually."

"'Eventually' might mean to-morrow morning"--drily--"and that would be just twelve hours too late. It's worth the risk fifty times over."

"It's not!"--passionately. "Do you suppose I care two straws for the gossip of a parcel of spiteful old women?"

"Not at the moment, perhaps, but later you wouldn't be able to help it. What people think of you, what they say of you, can make all the difference between heaven and hell." He spoke heavily, as though his words were weighted with some deadening memory. "And do you think I could bear to feel that I--*I* had given people a handle for gossiping about you? I'd cut their tongues out first!" he added savagely.

He stripped off his coat, and, sitting down on a rock, began removing his boots, while Sara stood watching him in silence with big, sombre eyes.

Presently he stood up, bareheaded and barefooted. Below the lean, tanned face the column of his throat showed white as a woman's, while the thin silk of his vest revealed the powerful line of shoulder at its base. His keen eyes were gazing steadily across to the opposite shore, as though measuring the distance he must traverse, and as a chance shaft from the westering sun rested upon him, investing him momentarily in its radiance, there seemed something rather splendid about him--something very sure and steadfast and utterly without fear.

A sharp cry broke from Sara.

"Garth! Garth!"--his name sprang to her lips spontaneously. "You mustn't go! You mustn't go! . . ."

He wheeled round, and at the sight of her white, strained face a sudden light leapt into his eyes--the light of a great incredulity with, back of it, an unutterable hope and longing. In two strides he was at her side, his hands gripping her shoulders.

"Why, Sara?--God in heaven!"--the words came hurrying from him, hoarse and uneven--"I believe you care!"

For an instant he hesitated, seeming to hold himself in check, then he caught her in his arms, kissing her fiercely on eyes and lips and throat.

"My dear! . . . Oh! My dear! . . ."

She could hear the broken words stammered through his hurried breathing as she lay unresistingly in his arms; then she felt him put her from him, gently, decisively, and she stood alone, swaying slightly. A long shuddering sigh ran through her body.

"Garth!"

She never knew whether the word really passed her lips or whether it was only the cry of her inmost being, so importunate, so urgent that it seemed to take on actual sound.

There came no answer. He was gone, and through the light veil of the encroaching mists she could see him shearing his way through the leaden-coloured sea.

She remained motionless, her eyes straining after him. He was swimming easily, with a powerful overhand stroke that carried him swiftly away from the shore. A little sigh of relaxed tension fluttered between her lips. At least, he was a magnificent swimmer--he had that much in his favour.

Then her glance spanned the channel to the further shore, and it seemed as though an interminable waste of water stretched between. And all the time, at every stroke, that mad, racing current was pulling against him, fighting for possession of the strong, sinewy body battling against it.

She beat her hands together in an agony of fear. Why had she let him go? What did it matter if people talked--what was a tarnished reputation to set against a man's life? Oh! She had been mad to let him go!

The fog grew denser. Strain as she might, she could no longer see the dark head above the water, the rise and fall of his arm like a white flail in the murky light, and she realized that should exhaustion overtake him, or the swift-running current beat him, drawing him under--she would not even know?

A sickening sense of bitter impotence assailed her. There was nothing she could do but wait--wait helplessly until either his return, or endless hours of solitude, told her whether he had won or lost the fight against that grey, hungry waste of water. A strangled sob burst from her throat.

"Oh, God! Let him come back to me! Let him come back!"

The creak of straining rowlocks and the even plash of dripping oars, muffled by the numbing curtain of the fog, broke through the silence. Then followed the gentle thudding noise of a boat as it bumped against the jetty and a voice--Garth's voice--calling.

She rose from the ground where she had flung herself and came to him, peering at him with eyes that looked like two dark stains in the whiteness of her face.

"I though you were dead," she said dully. "Drowned. I mean--oh, of course, it's the same thing, isn't it?" And she laughed, the shrill, choking laughter of overwrought nerves.

Garth observed her narrowly.

"No, I've very much alive, thanks," he said, speaking in deliberately cheerful and commonplace accents. "But you look half frozen. Why on earth didn't you put the rug round you? Get into the boat and let me tuck you up."

She obeyed passively, and in a few minutes they were slipping over the water as rapidly as the mist permitted.

Sara was very silent throughout the return journey. For hours, for an eternity it seemed, she had been in the grip of a consuming terror, culminating at last in the conviction that Garth had failed to make the further shore. And now, with the knowledge of his safety, the reaction from the tension of acute anxiety left her utterly flaccid and exhausted, incapable of anything more than a half-stunned acceptance of the miracle.

When at last the Selwyns' house was reached, it was with a manifest effort that she roused herself sufficiently to answer Garth's quiet apology for the misadventure of the afternoon.

"If it was your fault that we got stranded on the island," she said, summoning up rather a wan smile, "it is, at all events, thanks to you that I shall be sleeping under a respectable roof, instead of scandalizing half the neighbourhood!" She paused, then went on uncertainly: "'Thank you' seems ludicrously inadequate for all you've done--"

"I've done nothing," he interrupted brusquely.

"You risked your life--"

An impatient exclamation broke from him.

"And if I did? I risked something of no value, I assure you--to myself, or any one else."

Then he added practically--

"Get Jane Crab to give you some hot soup and go to bed. You look absolutely done."

Sara nodded, smiling more naturally.

"I will," she said. "Good-night, then." She held out her hand a little nervously.

He took it, holding it closely in his, and looking down at her with the strange expression of a man who strives to impress upon his mind the picture of a face he may not see again, so that in a lonely future he shall find comfort in remembering.

"Good-bye!" he said, at last, very gravely. Then a queer little smile, half-bitter, half-tender, curving his lips, he added: "I shall always have this one day for which to thank whatever gods there be."

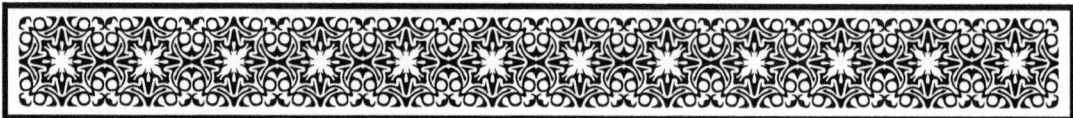

CHAPTER XII
A REVOKE

Sara lay long awake that night. Under Jane Crab's bluff and kindly ministrations, her feeling of utter bodily exhaustion had given place to an exquisite sense of mental and physical well-being, and, freed from the shackles of material discomfort, her thoughts flew backward over the events of the day.

All *was* well--gloriously, blessedly well! There could be no misunderstanding that brief, passionate moment when Garth had held her in his arms; and the blinding anguish of those hours which had followed, when she had not known whether he were alive or dead, had shown her her own heart.

Love had come to her--the love which Patrick Lovell had called the one altogether good and perfect gift--and with it came a tremulous unrest, a shy sweetness of desire that crept through all her veins like the burning of a swift flame.

She felt no fear or shame of love. Sara would never be afraid of life and its demands, and it seemed to her a matter of little moment that Garth had made no conventional avowal of his love. She did not, on that account, pretend, even to herself, as many women would have done, that her own heart was untouched, but recognized and accepted the fact that love had come to her with absolute simplicity.

Nor did she doubt or question Garth's feeling for her. She *knew*, in every fibre of her being, that he loved her, and she was ready to wait quite patiently and happily the few hours that must elapse before he could come to her and tell her so.

Yet she longed, with a woman's natural longing, to hear him say in actual words all that his whole attitude towards her had implied, craved for the moment when the beloved voice should ask for that surrender which in spirit she had already made.

She rose early, with a ridiculous feeling that it would bring the time a little nearer, and Jane Crab stared in amazement when she appeared downstairs while yet the preparations for breakfast were hardly in progress.

"You're no worse for your outing, then, Miss Tennant," she observed, adding shrewdly: "I'd as lief think you were the better for it."

Sara laughed, flushing a little. Somehow she did not mind the humorous suspicion of the truth that twinkled in Jane's small, boot-button eyes, but she sincerely hoped that the rest of the household would not prove equally discerning.

She need have had no fears on that score. Dr. Selwyn had barely time to swallow a cup of coffee and a slice of toast before rushing off in response to an urgent summons from a patient, whilst Molly seemed entirely preoccupied with the contents of a letter, in an unmistakably masculine handwriting, which had come for her by the morning's post. As for Mrs. Selwyn, she was always too much engrossed in analyzing the symptoms of some fresh ailment she believed she had acquired to be sensible of the emotional atmosphere of those around her. Her own sensations--whether she were too hot, or not quite hot enough, whether her new tabloids were suiting her or whether she had not slept as well as usual--occupied her entire horizon.

This morning she was distressed because the hairpins Sara had purchased for her the previous day differed slightly in shape from those she was in the habit of using.

Sara explained that they were the only ones obtainable.

"At Bloxham's, you mean, dear. Oh, well, of course, you couldn't get any others, then. Perhaps if you had tried another shop--" Mrs. Selwyn paused, to let this suggestion sink in, then added brightly: "But, naturally, I couldn't expect you to spend your whole morning going from shop to shop looking for my particular kind of hairpin, could I?"

Sara, who had expended a solid hour over that very occupation, was perfectly conscious of the reproach implied. She ignored it, however. Like every one else in close contact with Mrs. Selwyn, she had learned to accept the fact that the poor lady seriously believed that her whole life was spent in bearing with admirable patience the total absence of consideration accorded her.

When she descended from Mrs. Selwyn's room Sara was amazed to find that the hands of the clock only indicated half-past ten. Surely no morning had ever dragged itself away so slowly!

At two o'clock she and Molly were both due to lunch with Mrs. Maynard at Greenacres, and she was radiantly aware that Garth Trent would be included among the guests. Between them, Audrey, and the Herricks, and Sara had succeeded in enticing the hermit within the charmed circle of their friendship, and he could now be depended upon to join their little gatherings--"provided," as he had bluntly told Audrey, "that you can put up with my manners and morals."

Mrs. Maynard had only laughed.

"I'm not in the least likely to find fault with your manners," she said cheerfully. "They're really quite normal, and as for your morals, they are your own affair, my dear man. Anyway, there is at least one bond between us--Monkshaven heartily disapproves of both of us."

Greenacres was a delightful place, built rather on the lines of a French country house, with the sitting-rooms leading one into the other and each opening in its turn on to a broad wooden verandah. The latter ran round three sides of the house, and in summer the delicate pink of Dorothy Perkins fought for supremacy with the deeper red of the Crimson Rambler, converting it into a literal bower of roses.

Audrey was on the steps to greet the two girls when they arrived, looking, as usual, as though she had just quitted the hands of an expert French maid. It was in a great measure to the ultra-perfection of her toilette that she owed the critical attitude accorded her by the feminine half of Monkshaven. To the provincial mind, the fact that she dyed her hair, ordered her frocks from Paris, and kept a French chef to cook her food, were all so many indications of an altogether worldly and abandoned character--and of a wealth that was secretly to be envied--and the more venomous among Audrey's detractors lived in the perennial hope of some day unveiling the scandal which they were convinced lay hidden in her past.

Audrey was perfectly aware of the gossip of which she was the subject--and completely indifferent to it.

"It amuses them," she would say blithely, "and it doesn't hurt me in the least. If Mr. Trent and I both left the neighbourhood, Monkshaven would be at a loss for a topic of conversation--unless they decided, as they probably would, that we had eloped together!"

She herself was quite above the petty meanness of envying another woman's looks or clothes, and she beamed frank admiration over Molly's appearance as she led the way into the house.

"Molly, you're too beautiful to be true," she declared, pausing in the hall to inspect the girl's young loveliness in its setting of shady hat and embroidered muslin frock. Big golden poppies on the hat, and a girdle at her waist of the same tawny hue, emphasized the rare colour of her eyes--in shadow, brown like an autumn leaf, gold like amber when the sunlight lay in them--and the whole effect was deliciously arresting.

"You've been spending your substance in riotous purple and fine linen," pursued Audrey relentlessly. "That frock was never evolved in Oldhampton, I'm positive."

Molly blushed--not the dull, unbecoming red most women achieve, but a delicate pink like the inside of a shell that made her look even more irresistibly distracting than before.

"No," she admitted reluctantly, "I sent for this from town."

Sara glanced at her with quick surprise. Entirely absorbed in her own thoughts, she had failed to observe the expensive charm of Molly's toilette and now regarded it attentively. Where had she obtained the money to pay for it? Only a very little while ago she had been in debt, and now here she was launching out into expenditure which common sense would suggest must be quite beyond her means.

Sara frowned a little, but, recognizing the impossibility of probing into the matter at the moment, she dismissed it from her mind, resolving to elucidate the mystery later on.

Meanwhile, it was impossible to do other than acknowledge the results obtained. Molly looked more like a stately young empress than an impecunious doctor's daughter as she floated into the room, to be embraced and complimented by the Lavender Lady and to receive a generous meed of admiration, seasoned with a little gentle banter, from Miles Herrick.

Sara experienced a sensation of relief on discovering Miss Lavinia and Herrick to be the only occupants of the room. Garth Trent had not yet come. Despite her longing to see him again, she was conscious of a certain diffidence, a reluctance at meeting him in the presence of others, and she wished fervently that their first meeting after the events of the previous day could have taken place anywhere rather than at this gay little lunch party of Audrey's.

As it fell out, however, she chanced to be entirely alone in the room when Trent was at length ushered in by a trim maidservant, the rest of the party having gradually drifted out on to the verandah, while she had lingered behind, glad of a moment's solitude in which to try and steady herself.

She had never conceived it possible that so commonplace an emotion as mere nervousness could find place beside the immensities of love itself, yet, during the interminable moment when Garth crossed the room to her side, she was supremely aware of an absurd desire to turn and flee, and it was only by a sheer effort of will that she held her ground.

The next moment he had shaken hands with her and was making some tranquil observation upon the lateness of his arrival. His manner was quite detached, every vestige of anything beyond mere conventional politeness banished from it.

The coolly neutral inflections of his voice struck upon Sara's keyed-up consciousness as an indifferent finger may twang the stretched strings of a violin, producing a shuddering violation of their harmony.

She hardly knew how she answered him. She only knew, with a sudden overwhelming certainty, that the Garth who stood beside her now was a different man, altered out of all kinship with the man who had held her in his arms on Devil's Hood Island. The lover was gone; only the acquaintance remained.

She stammered a few halting words by way of response, and--was she mistaken, or did a sudden look of understanding, almost, it seemed, of compunction, leap for a moment into his eyes, only to be replaced by the brooding, bitter indifference habitual to them?

The opportune return of Audrey and her other guests, heralded by a gust of cheerful laughter, tided over the difficult moment, and Garth turned away to make his apologies to his hostess, blaming some slight mishap to his car for the tardiness of his appearance.

Throughout lunch Sara conversed mechanically, responding like an automaton when any one put a penny in the slot by asking her a question. She felt utterly bewildered, stunned by Garth's behaviour.

Had their meeting been exchanged under the observant eyes of the rest of the party, it would have been intelligible to her, for he was the last man in the world to wear his heart upon his sleeve. But they had been quite alone for the moment, and yet he had permitted no acknowledgment of the new relations between them to appear either in word or look. He had greeted her precisely as though they were no more to each other than the merest acquaintances--as though the happenings of the previous day had been wiped out of his mind. It was incomprehensible!

Sara felt almost as if some one had dealt her a physical blow, and it required all her pluck and poise to enable her to take her share of the general conversation before wending their several ways homeward.

". . . And we'll picnic on Devil's Hood Island."

Audrey's high, clear voice, as she chattered to Molly, characteristically propounding half-a-dozen plans for the immediate future, floated across to Sara where she stood waiting on the lowest step, impatient to be gone. As though drawn by some invisible magnet, her eyes encountered Garth's, and the swift colour rushed into her cheeks, staining them scarlet.

His expression was enigmatical. The next moment he bent forward and spoke, in a low voice that reached her ear alone.

"Much maligned place--where I tasted my one little bit of heaven!" Then, after a pause, he added deliberately: "But a black sheep has no business with heaven. He'd be turned away from the doors--and quite rightly, too! That's why I shall never ask for admittance." He regarded her steadily for a moment, then quietly averted his eyes.

And Sara realized that in those few words he had revoked--repudiating all that he had claimed, all that he had given, the day before.

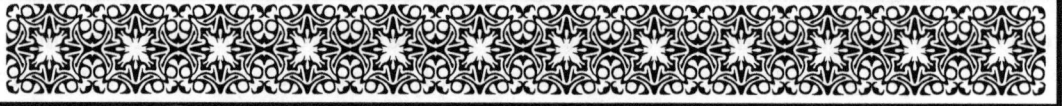

CHAPTER XIII
DISILLUSION

Letters are unsatisfactory things at the best of times, and what we all want is to have you with us again for a little while. I am sure you must have had a surfeit of the simple life by this time, so come to us and be luxurious and exotic in London for a change. Don't disappoint us, Sara!

"Yours ever affectionately,

"ELISABETH."

Sara, seated at the open window of her room, re-read the last paragraph of the letter which the morning's post had brought her, and then let it fall again on to her lap, whilst she stared with sombre eyes across the bay to where the Monk's Cliff reared itself, stark and menacing, against the sky.

April had slipped into May, and the blue waters of the Channel flickered with a myriad dancing points of light reflected from an unclouded sun. The trees had clothed themselves anew in pale young green, and the whole atmosphere was redolent of spring--spring as she reaches her maturity before she steps aside to let the summer in.

Sara frowned a little. She was out of tune with the harmony of things. You need happiness in your heart to be at one with the eager pulsing of new life, the reaching out towards fulfillment that is the essential quality of spring. Whereas Sara's heart was empty of happiness and hopes, and of all the joyous beginnings that are the glorious appanage of youth. There could be no beginnings for her, because she had already reached the end--reached it with such a stupefying suddenness that for a time she had been hardly conscious of pain, but only of a fierce, intolerable resentment and of a pride--that "devil's own pride" which Patrick had told her was the Tennant heritage--which had been wounded to the quick.

Garth had taken that pride of hers and ground it under his heel. He had played at love, and she had been fool enough to mistake love's simulacrum for the real thing. Or, if there had been any genuine spark of love kindling the fire of passion that had blazed about her for one brief moment, then he had since chosen deliberately to disavow it.

He had indicated his intention unmistakably. Since the day of the luncheon party at Greenacres he had shunned meeting her whenever possible, and, on the one or two occasions when an encounter had been unavoidable, his manner had been frigidly indifferent and impersonal.

Outwardly she had repaid him in full measure--indifference for indifference, ice for ice, gallantly matching her woman's pride against his deliberate apathy, but inwardly she writhed at the remembrance of that day on the island, when, in the stress of her terror for his safety, she had let him see into the very heart of her.

Well, it was over now, and done with. The brief vision of love which had given a new, transcendent significance to the whole of life, had faded swiftly into bleak darkness, its memory marred by that bitterest of all knowledge to a woman--the knowledge that she had been willing to give her love, to make the great surrender, and that it had not been required of her. All that remained was to draw a veil as decently as might be over the forgettable humiliation.

The strain of the last fortnight had left its mark on her. The angles of her face seemed to have become more sharply defined, and her eyes were too brilliant and held a look of restlessness. But her lips closed as firmly as ever, a courageous scarlet line, denying the power of fate to thrust her under.

The Book of Garth--the book of love--was closed, but there were many other volumes in life's library, and Sara did not propose to go through the probable remaining fifty or sixty years of her existence uselessly bewailing a dead past. She would face life, gamely, whatever it might bring, and as she had already sustained one of the hardest blows ever likely to befall her, she would probably make a success of it.

But, unquestionably, she would be glad to get away from Monkshaven for a time, to have leisure to readjust her outlook on life, free from the ceaseless reminders that the place held for her.

Here in Monkshaven, it seemed as though Garth's personality informed the very air she breathed. The great cliff where he had his dwelling frowned at her from across the bay whenever she looked out of her window, his name was constantly on the lips of those who made up her little circle of friends, and every day she was haunted by the fear of meeting him. Or, worse than all else, should that fear materialize, the torment of the almost hostile relationship which had replaced their former friendship had to be endured.

The invitation to join the Durwards in London had come at an opportune moment, offering, as it did, a way of escape from the embarrassments inseparable from the situation. Moreover, amid the distractions and bustle of the great city it would be easier to forget for a little her burden of pain and humiliation. There is so much time for thinking--and for remembering--in the leisurely tranquillity of country life.

Sara would have accepted the invitation without hesitation, but that there seemed to her certain reasons why her absence from Sunnyside just now was inadvisable--reasons based on her loyalty to Doctor Dick and the trust he had reposed in her.

For the last few weeks she had been perplexed and not a little worried concerning Molly's apparent accession to comparative wealth. Certain small extravagances in which the latter had recently indulged must have been, Sara knew, beyond the narrow limits of her purse, and inquiry had elicited from Selwyn the fact that she had received no addition to her usual allowance.

Molly herself had light-heartedly evaded all efforts to gain her confidence, and Sara had refrained from putting any direct question, since, after all, she was not the girl's guardian, and her interference might very well be resented.

She was uneasily conscious that for some reason or other Molly was in a state of tension, alternating between abnormally high spirits and the depths of depression, and the recollection of that unpleasant little episode of her indebtedness to Lester Kent lingered disagreeably in Sara's mind.

She had seen the man once, in Oldhampton High Street--Molly, at that time still clothed in penitence, had pointed him out to her--and she had received an unpleasing impression of a lean, hatchet face with deep-set, dense-brown eyes, and of a mouth like that of a bird of prey.

She felt reluctant to go away and leave things altogether to chance, and finally, unable to come to any decision, she carried Elisabeth's letter down to Selwyn's study and explained the position.

His face clouded over at the prospect of her departure.

"We shall miss you abominably," he declared. "But of course"--ruefully--"I can quite understand Mrs. Durward's wanting you to go back to them for a time, and I suppose we must resign ourselves to being unselfish. Only you must promise to come back again--you mustn't desert us altogether."

She laughed.

"You needn't be afraid of that. I shall turn up again like the proverbial bad penny."

"All the same, make it a promise," he urged.

"I promise, then, you distrustful man! But about Molly?"

"I don't think you need worry about her." Selwyn laughed a little. "The sudden accession to wealth is accounted for. It seems that she has sold a picture."

"Oh! So that's the explanation, is it?" Sara felt unaccountably relieved.

"Yes--though goodness knows how she has beguiled any one into buying one of her daubs!"

"Oh, they're quite good, really, Doctor Dick. It's only that Futurist Art doesn't appeal to you."

"Not exactly! She showed me one of her paintings the other day. It looked like a bad motor-bus accident in a crowded street, and she told me that it represented the physical atmosphere of a woman who had just been jilted."

Sara laughed suddenly and hysterically.

"How--how awfully funny!" she said in an odd, choked voice. Then, fearful of losing her self-command, she added hastily: "I'll write and tell Elisabeth that I'll come, then." And fled out of the room.

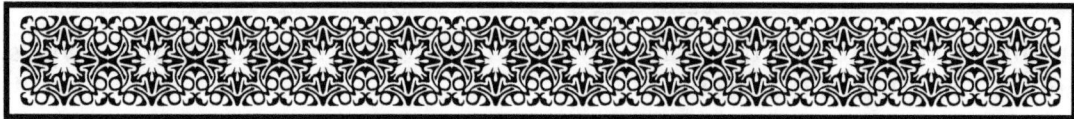

CHAPTER XIV
ELISABETH INTERVENES

As Sara stepped out of the train at Paddington, the first person upon whom her eyes alighted was Tim Durward. He hastened up to her.

"Tim!" she exclaimed delightedly. "How dear of you to come and meet me!"

"Didn't you expect I should?" He was holding her hand and joyfully pump-handling it up and down as though he would never let it go, while the glad light in his eyes would indubitably have betrayed him to any passer-by who had chanced to glance in his direction.

Sara coloured faintly and withdrew her hands from his eager clasp.

"Oh, well, you might conceivably have had something else to do," she returned evasively.

For an instant the blue eyes clouded.

"I never had anything to do," he said shortly. "You know that."

She laughed up at him.

"Now, Tim, I won't be growled at the first minute of my arrival. You can pour out your grumbles another day. First now, I want to hear all the news. Remember, I've been vegetating in the country since the beginning of March!"

She drew him tactfully away from the old sore subject of his enforced idleness, and, while the car bore them swiftly towards the Durwards' house on Green Street, she entertained him with a description of the Selwyn trio.

"I should think your 'Doctor Dick' considers himself damned lucky in having got you there--seeing that his house seems all at sixes and sevens," commented Tim rather glumly.

"He does. Oh! I'm quite appreciated, I assure you."

Tim made no reply, but stared out of the window. The car rounded the corner into Park Lane; in another moment they would reach their destination. Suddenly he turned to her, his face rather strained-looking.

"And--the other man? Have you met him yet--at Monkshaven?"

There was no mistaking his meaning. Sara's eyes met his unflinchingly.

"If you mean has any one asked me to marry him--no, Tim. No one has done me that honour," she answered lightly.

"Thank God!" he muttered below his breath.

Sara looked troubled.

"Haven't you--got over that, yet?" she said, hesitatingly. "I--I hoped you would, Tim."

"I shall never get over it," he asserted doggedly. "And I shall never give you up till you are another man's wife."

The quiet intensity of his tones sounded strangely in her ears. This was a new Tim, not the boyish Tim of former times, but a man with all a man's steadfast purpose and determination.

She was spared the necessity of reply by the fact that they had reached their journey's end. The car slid smoothly to a standstill, and almost simultaneously the house-door opened, and behind the immaculate figure of the Durwards' butler Sara descried the welcoming faces of Geoffrey and Elisabeth.

It was good to see them both again--Geoffrey, big and debonair as ever, his jolly blue eyes beaming at her delightedly, and Elisabeth, still with that same elusive atmosphere of charm which always seemed to cling about her like the fragrance of a flower.

They were eager to hear Sara's news, plying her with questions, so that before the end of her first evening with them they had gleaned a fairly accurate description of her life at Sunnyside and of the new circle of friends she had acquired.

But there was one name she refrained from mentioning--that of Garth Trent, and none of Elisabeth's quietly uttered comments or inquiries sufficed to break through the guard of her reticence concerning the Hermit of Far End.

"It sounds rather a manless Eden--except for the nice, lame Herrick person," said Elisabeth at last, and her hyacinth eyes, with their curiously veiled expression, rested consideringly on Sara's face, alight with interest as she had vividly sketched the picture of her life at Monkshaven.

"Yes, I suppose it is rather," she admitted. Her tone was carelessly indifferent, but the eager light died suddenly out of her face, and Elisabeth, smiling faintly, adroitly turned the conversation.

Sara speedily discovered that she would have even less time for the fruitless occupation of remembering than she had anticipated. The Durwards owned a host of friends in town with whom they were immensely popular, and Sara found herself caught up in a perpetual whirl of entertainment that left her but little leisure for brooding over the past.

She felt sometimes as though the London season had opened and swallowed her up, as the whale swallowed Jonah, and when she declared herself breathless with so much rushing about, Tim would coolly throw over any engagement that chanced to have been made and carry her off for a day up the river, where a quiet little lunch, in the tranquil shade of overhanging trees, and the cosy, intimate talk that was its invariable concomitant, seemed like an oasis of familiar, homely pleasantness in the midst of the gay turmoil of London in May.

Tim had developed amazingly. He seemed instinctively to recognize her moods, adapting himself accordingly, and in his thought and care for her there was a half-playful, half-tender element of possessiveness that sometimes brought a smile to her lips--and sometimes a sigh, as the inevitable comparison asserted itself between Tim's gentle ruling and the brusque, forceful mastery that had been Garth's. But, on the whole, the visit to the Durwards was productive of more smiles than sighs, and Sara found Tim's young, chivalrous devotion very soothing to the wound her pride had suffered at Garth's hands.

She overflowed in gratitude to Elisabeth.

"You're giving me a perfectly lovely time," she told her. "And Tim *is* such a good playfellow!"

Elisabeth's face seemed suddenly to glow with that inner radiance which praise of her beloved Tim alone was able to inspire.

"Only that, Sara?" she said very quietly. Yet somehow Sara knew that she meant to have an answer to her question.

"Why--why----" she stammered a little. "Isn't that enough?"--trying to speak lightly.

Elisabeth shook her head.

"Tim wants more than a playfellow. Can't you give him what he wants, Sara?"

Sara was silent a moment.

"I didn't know he had told you," she said, at last, rather lamely.

"Nor has he. Tim is loyal to the core. But a mother doesn't need telling these things." Elisabeth's beautiful voice deepened. "Tim is bone of my bone and flesh of my flesh--and he's soul of my soul as well. Do you think, then, that I shouldn't know when he is hurt?"

Sara was strangely moved. There was something impressive in the restrained passion of Elisabeth's speech, a certain primitive grandeur in her envisagement of the relationship of mother and son.

"I expect," pursued Elisabeth calmly, "that you think I'm going too far--farther than I have any right to. But it's any mother's right to fight for her son's happiness, and I'm fighting for Tim's. Why won't you marry him, Sara?" The question flashed out suddenly.

"Because--why--oh, because I'm not in love with him."

A gleam of rather sardonic mirth showed in Elisabeth's face.

"I wish," she observed, "that we lived in the good old days when you could have been carried off by sheer force and *compelled* to marry him."

Sara laughed outright.

"I really believe you mean it!" she said with some amusement.

Elisabeth nodded.

"I do. I shouldn't have hesitated."

"And what about me? You wouldn't have considered my feelings at all in the matter, I suppose?" Sara was still smiling, yet she had a dim consciousness that, preposterous as it sounded, Elisabeth would have had no scruples whatever about putting such a plan into effect had it been in any way feasible.

"No." Elisabeth replied with the utmost composure. "Tim comes first. But"--and suddenly her voice melted to an indescribable sweetness--"You would be almost one with him in my heart, because you had brought him happiness." She paused, then launched her question with a delicate hesitancy that skillfully concealed all semblance of the probe. "Tell me--is there any one else who has asked of you what Tim asks? Perhaps I have come too late with my plea?"

Sara shook her head.

"No," she said flatly, "there is no one else." With a sudden bitter self-mockery she added: "Tim's is the only proposal of marriage I have to my credit."

The repressed anxiety with which Elisabeth had been regarding her relaxed, and a curious look of content took birth in the hyacinth eyes. It was as though the bitterness of Sara's answer in some way reassured her, serving her purpose.

"Then can't you give Tim what he wants? You will be robbing no one. Sara"-- her low voice vibrated with the urgency of her desire--"promise me at least that you will think it over--that you will not dismiss the idea as though it were impossible?"

Sara half rose; her eyes, wide and questioning, were fixed upon Elisabeth's.

"But why--why do you ask me this?" she faltered.

"Because I think"--very softly--"that Tim himself will ask you the same thing before very long. And I can't face what it will mean to him if you send him away. . . . You would be happy with him, Sara. No woman could live with Tim and not grow to love him--certainly no woman whom Tim loved."

The depth of her conviction imbued her words with a strange force of suggestion. For the first time the idea of marriage with Tim presented itself to Sara as a remotely conceivable happening.

Hitherto she had looked upon his love for her as something which only touched the outer fringe of her life--a temporary disturbance of the good-comradely relations that had existed between them. With the easy optimism of a woman whose heart has always been her own exclusive property she had hoped he would "get over it."

But now Elisabeth's appeal, and the knowledge of the pain of love, which love itself had taught her, quickened her mind to a new understanding. Perhaps Elisabeth felt her yield to the impression she had been endeavoring to create, for she rose and came and stood quite close to her, looking down at her with shining eyes.

"Give my son his happiness!" she said. And the eternal supplication of all motherhood was in her voice.

Sara made no answer. She sat very still, with bent head. Presently there came the sound of light footsteps as Elisabeth crossed the room, and, a moment later, the door closed softly behind her.

She had thrust a new responsibility on Sara's shoulders--the responsibility of

Tim's happiness.

"Give my son his happiness!" The poignant appeal of the words rang in Sara's ears.

After all, why not? As Elisabeth had said, she would be robbing no one by so doing. The man for whom had been reserved the place in the sacred inner temple of her heart had signified very clearly that he had no intention of claiming it.

No other would ever enter in his stead; the doors of that innermost sanctuary would be kept closed, shutting in only the dead ashes of remembrance. But if entrance to the outer courts of the temple meant so much to Tim, why should she not make him free of them? That other had come and gone again, having no need of her, while Tim's need was great.

Life, at the moment stretched in front of her very vague and purposeless, and she knew that by marrying Tim she would make three people whom she loved, and who mattered most to her in the whole world--Tim, and Elisabeth, and Geoffrey--supremely happy. No one need suffer except herself--and for her there was no escape from suffering either way.

So it came about that when, as her visit drew towards its close, Tim came to her and asked her once again to be his wife, she gave him an answer which by no stretch of the imagination could she have conceived as possible a short three weeks before.

She was very frank with him. She was determined that if he married her, it must be open-eyed, recognizing that she could only give him honest liking in return for love. Upon a foundation of sincerity some mutual happiness might ultimately be established, but there should be no submerged rock of ignorance and misunderstanding on which their frail barque of matrimonial happiness might later founder in a sea of infinite regret.

"Are you willing to take me--like that?" she asked him. "Knowing that I can only give you friendship? I wish--I wish I could give you what you ask--but I can't."

Tim's eyes searched hers for a long moment.

"Is there some one else?" he asked at last.

A wave of painful colour flooded her face, then ebbed away, leaving it curiously white and pinched-looking, but her eyes still met his bravely.

"There is--no one who will ever want your place, Tim," she said with an effort.

The sight of her evident distress hurt him intolerably.

"Forgive me!" he exclaimed quickly. "I had no right to ask that question."

"Yes, you had," she replied steadily, "since you have asked me to be your wife."

"Well, you've answered it--and it doesn't make a bit of difference. I want you. I'll take what you can give me, Sara. Perhaps, some day, you'll be able to give me love as well."

She shook her head.

"Don't count on that, Tim. Friendship, understanding, the comradeship which, after all, can mean a good deal between a man and woman--all these I can give you. And if you think those things are worth while, I'll marry you. But--I'm not in love with you."

"You will be--I'm sure it's catching," he declared with the gay, buoyant confidence which was one of his most endearing qualities.

Sara smiled a little wistfully.

"I wish it were," she said. "But please be serious, Tim dear--"

"How can I be?" he interrupted joyfully. "When the woman I love tells me that she'll marry me, do you suppose I'm going to pull a long face about it?"

He caught her in his arms and kissed her with all the impetuous fervour of his two-and-twenty years. At the touch of his warm young lips, her own lips whitened. For an instant, as she rested in his arms, she was stabbed through and through by the memory of those other arms that had held her as in a vice of steel, and of stormy, passionate kisses in comparison with Tim's impulsive caress, half-shy, half-reverent, seemed like clear water beside the glowing fire of red wine.

She drew herself sharply out of his embrace. Would she never forget--would she be for ever remembering, comparing? If so, God help her!

"No," she said quietly. "You needn't pull a long face over it. But--but marriage is a serious thing, Tim, after all."

"My dear"--he spoke with a sudden gentle gravity--"don't misunderstand me. Marriage with you is the most serious and wonderful and glorious thing that could ever happen to a man. When you're my wife, I shall be thanking God on my knees every day of my life. All the jokes and nonsense are only so many little waves of happiness breaking on the shore. But behind them there is always the big sea of my love for you--the still waters, Sara."

Sara remained silent. The realization of the tender, chivalrous, worshiping love this boy was pouring out at her feet made her feel very humble--very ashamed and sorry that she could give so little in return.

Presently she turned and held out her hands to him.

"Tim--my Tim," she said, and her voice shook a little. "I'll try not to disappoint you."

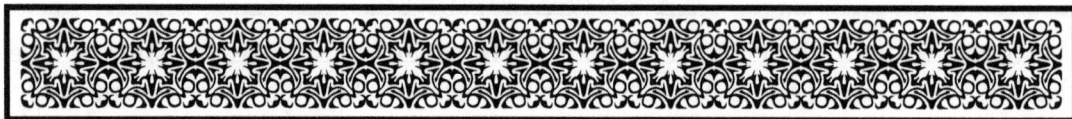

CHAPTER XV
THE NAME OF DURWARD

The Durwards received the news of their son's engagement to Sara with unfeigned delight. Geoffrey was bluffly gratified at the materialization of his private hopes, and Elisabeth had never appeared more captivating than during the few days that immediately followed. She went about as softly radiant and content as a pleased child, and even the strange, watchful reticence that dwelt habitually in her eyes was temporarily submerged by the shining happiness that welled up within them.

She urged that an early date should be fixed for the wedding, and Sara, with a dreary feeling that nothing really mattered very much, listlessly acquiesced. Driven by conflicting influences she had burned her boats, and the sooner all signs of the conflagration were obliterated the better.

But she opposed a quiet negative to the further suggestion that she should accompany the Durwards to Barrow Court instead of returning to Monkshaven.

"No, I can't do that," she said with decision. "I promised Doctor Dick I would go back."

Elisabeth smiled airily. Apparently she had no scruples about the keeping of promises.

"That's easily arranged," she affirmed. "I'll write to your precious doctor man and tell him that we can't spare you."

As far as personal inclination was concerned, Sara would gladly have adopted Elisabeth's suggestion. She shrank inexpressibly from returning to Monkshaven, shrouded, as it was, in brief but poignant memories, but she had given Selwyn her word that she would go back, and, even in a comparatively unimportant matter such as this appeared, she had a predilection in favour of abiding by a promise.

Elisabeth demurred.

"You're putting Dr. Selwyn before us," she declared, candidly amazed.

"I promised him first," replied Sara. "In my position, you'd do the same."

Elisabeth shook her head.

"I shouldn't," she replied with energy. "The people I love come first--all the rest nowhere."

"Then I'm glad I'm one of the people you love," retorted Sara, laughing. "And, let me tell you, I think you're a most unmoral person."

Elisabeth looked at her reflectively.

"Perhaps I am," she acknowledged. "At least, from a conventional point of view. Certainly I shouldn't let any so-called moral scruples spoil the happiness of any one I cared about. However, I suppose you would, and so we're all to be offered up on the altar of this twopenny-halfpenny promise you've made to Dr. Selwyn?"

Sara laughed and kissed her.

"I'm afraid you are," she said.

If anything could have reconciled her to the sacrifice of inclination she had made in returning to Monkshaven, it would have been the warmth of the welcome extended to her on her arrival. Selwyn and Molly met her at the station, and Jane Crab, resplendent in a new cap and apron donned for the occasion, was at the gate when at last the pony brought the governess-cart to a standstill outside. Even Mrs. Selwyn had exerted herself to come downstairs, and was waiting in the hall to greet the wanderer back.

"It will be a great comfort to have you back, my dear," she said with unwonted feeling in her voice, and quite suddenly Sara felt abundantly rewarded for the many weary hours upstairs, trying to win Mrs. Selwyn's interest to anything exterior to herself.

"You're looking thinner," was Selwyn's blunt comment, as Sara threw off her hat and coat. "What have you been doing with yourself?"

She flushed a little.

"Oh, racketing about, I suppose. I've been living in a perfect whirl. Never mind, Doctor Dick, you shall fatten me up now with your good country food and your good country air. Good gracious!"--as he closed a big thumb and finger around her slender wrist and shook his head disparagingly--"Don't look so solemn! I was always one of the lean kine, you know."

"I don't think that London has agreed with you," rumbled Selwyn discontent-edly. "Your pulse is as jerky as a primitive cinema film. You'd better not be in such a hurry to run away from us again. Besides, we can't do without you, my dear."

With a mental jolt Sara recollected the fact of her approaching marriage. How on earth should she break it to these good friends of hers, who counted so much on her remaining with them, that within three months--the longest period Elisabeth would consent to wait--she would be leaving them permanently? It was manifestly impossible to pour such a douche of cold water into the midst of the joyful warmth of their welcome; and she decided to wait, at least until the next day, before ac-quainting them with the fact of her engagement.

When morning came, the same arguments held good in favour of a further postponement, and, as the days slipped by, it became increasingly difficult to intro-duce the subject.

Moreover, amid the change of environment and influence, Sara experienced a certain almost inevitable reaction of feeling. It was not that she actually regret-ted her engagement, but none the less she found herself supersensitively conscious of it, and she chafed against the thought of the congratulations and all the kindly, well-meant "fussation" which its announcement would entail.

She told herself irritably that this was only because she had not yet had time to get used to the idea of regarding herself as Tim's future wife; that, later on, when she had grown more accustomed to it, the prospect of her friends' felicitations would appear less repugnant. She had to face the ultimate fact that marriage, for her, did not mean the crowning fulfillment of life; marriage with Tim would never be any-thing more than a substitute, a next best thing.

With these thoughts in her mind, she finally decided to say nothing about her engagement for the present, but to pick up the threads of life at Sunnyside as though that crowded month in London, with its unexpected culmination, had never been.

Once taken, the decision afforded her a curious sense of respite and relief. It was very pleasant to drop back into the old habits of managing the Sunnyside *me-nage*--making herself indispensable to Selwyn, humouring his wife, and keeping a watchful eye on Molly.

The latter, Sara found, was by far the most difficult part of her task, and the vague apprehensions she had formed, and to some extent shared with Selwyn before her visit to London, increased.

From an essentially lovable, inconsequent creature, with a temper of an angel and the frankness of a child, Molly had become oddly nervous and irritable, flushing and paling suddenly for no apparent cause, and guardedly uncommunicative as to her comings and goings. She was oddly resentful of any manifestation of interest in her affairs, and snubbed Sara roundly when the latter ventured an injudicious inquiry as to whether Lester Kent were still in the neighbourhood.

"How on earth should I know?" The golden-brown eyes met Sara's with a look of nervous defiance. "I'm not his keeper." Then, as though slightly ashamed of her outburst, she added more amiably: "I haven't been down to the Club for weeks. It's been so hot--and I suppose I've been lazy. But I'm going to-morrow. I shall be able to gratify your curiosity concerning Lester Kent when I come home."

"To-morrow?" Sara looks surprised. "But we promised to go to tea with Audrey to-morrow."

Molly flushed and looked away.

"Did we?" she said vaguely. "I'd forgotten."

"Can't you arrange to go to Oldhampton the next day instead?" continued Sara.

Molly frowned a little. At last--

"I tell you what I'll do," she said agreeably. "I'll come back by the afternoon train and meet you at Greenacres." And with this concession Sara had to be content.

Tea at Greenacres resolved itself into a kind of rarefied picnic, and, as Sara crossed the cool green lawns in the wake of a smart parlourmaid, she found that quite a considerable number of Audrey's friends--and enemies--were gathered together under the shade of the trees, partaking of tea and strawberries and cream. The *elite* of the neighbourhood might find many disagreeable things to say concerning Mrs. Maynard, but they were not in the least averse to accepting her hospitality whenever the opportunity presented itself.

Sara's heart leapt suddenly as she descried Trent's lean, well-knit figure amongst those dotted about on the lawn. She had tried very hard to accustom herself to meet him with composure, but at each encounter, although outwardly quite cool, her pulses raced, and to-day, the first time she had seen him since her return from London, she felt as though all her nerves were outside her skin instead of underneath it.

He was talking to Miles Herrick. The latter, lying back luxuriously in a deck-chair, proceeded to wave and beckon an enthusiastic greeting as soon as he caught sight of Sara, and rather reluctantly she responded to his signals and made her way towards the two men.

"I feel like a bloated sultan summoning one of the ladies of the harem to his presence," confessed Miles apologetically when he had shaken hands. "I've added a sprained ankle to my other disabilities," he continued cheerfully. "Hence my apparent laziness."

Sara commiserated appropriately.

"How did you manage to get here?" she asked.

Miles gestured towards Trent.

"This man maintained that it was bad for my mental and moral health to brood alone at home while Lavinia went skipping off into society unchaperoned. So he fetched me along in his car."

Sara's eyes rested thoughtfully on Trent's face a moment.

It was odd how kindly and considerate he always showed himself towards Miles Herrick. Perhaps somewhere within him a responsive chord was touched by the evidence of the other man's broken life.

"Miss Tennant is thinking that it's a case of the blind leading the blind for me to act as a cicerone into society," remarked Trent curtly.

Sara winced at the repellent hardness of his tone, but she declined to take up the challenge.

"I am very glad you persuaded Miles to come over," was all she said.

Trent's lips closed in a straight line. It seemed as though he were trying to resist the appeal of her gently given answer; and Miles, conscious of the antagonism in the atmosphere, interposed with some commonplace question concerning her visit to London.

"You're looking thinner than you were, Sara," he added critically.

She flushed a little as she felt Trent's hawk-like glance sweep over her.

"Oh, I've been leading too gay a life," she said hastily. "The Durwards seem to know half London, so that we crowded about a dozen engagements into each day-- and a few more into the night."

"*Durward?*" The word sprang violently from Trent's lips, almost as though jerked out of him, and Sara, glancing towards him in some astonishment, surprised a strange, suddenly vigilant expression in his face. It was immediately succeeded by a blank look of indifference, yet beneath the assumption of indifference his eyes seemed to burn with a kind of slumbering hostility.

"Yes--the people I have been staying with," she explained. "Do you know them, by any chance?"

"I really can't say," he replied carelessly. "Durward is not a very uncommon name, is it?"

"Their name was originally Lovell--they only acquired the Durward with some property. Mrs. Durward is an extraordinarily beautiful woman. I believe in her younger days she had half London in love with her."

Sara hardly knew why she felt impelled to supply so many particulars concerning the Durwards. After that first brief exclamation, Trent seemed to have lost interest, and appeared to be rather bored by the recital than otherwise. He made no comment when she had finished.

"Then you don't know them?" she asked at last.

"I?" He started slightly, as though recalled to the present by her question. "No. I haven't the pleasure to be numbered amongst Mrs. Durward's friends," he said quietly. "I have seen her, however."

"She is very beautiful, don't you think?" persisted Sara.

"Very," he replied indifferently. And then, quite deliberately, he directed the conversation into another channel, leaving Sara feeling exactly as though a door had been slammed in her face.

It was his old method of putting an end to a discussion that failed to please him--this arrogantly abrupt transition to another subject--and, though it served its immediate purpose, it was a method that had its weaknesses. If you deliberately hide behind a hedge, any one who catches you in the act naturally wonders why you are doing it.

Even Miles looked a trifle astonished at Trent's curt dismissal of the Durward topic, and Sara, who had observed the strange expression that leaped into his eyes-- half-guarded, half inimical--felt convinced that he knew more about the Durwards than he had chosen to acknowledge.

She could not imagine in what way they were connected with his life, nor why he should have been so averse to admitting his knowledge of them. But there were many inexplicable circumstances associated with the man who had chosen to live more or less the life of a recluse at Far End; and Sara, and the little circle of intimates who had at last succeeded in drawing him into their midst, had accustomed themselves to the atmosphere of secrecy that seemed to envelope him.

From his obvious desire to eschew the society of his fellow men and women, and from the acid cynicism of his outlook on things in general, it had been gradually assumed amongst them that some happenings in the past had marred his life, poisoning the springs of faith, and hope, and charity at their very fount, and with the tact of real friendship they never sought to discover what he so evidently wished concealed.

"Where is Molly to-day?" Miles's pleasant voice broke across the awkward moment, giving yet a fresh trend to the conversation that was languishing uncomfortably.

Sara's gaze ranged searchingly over the little groups of people sprinkled about the lawn.

"Isn't she here yet?" she asked, startled. "She was coming back from Oldhampton by the afternoon train, and promised to meet me here."

Miles looked at his watch.

"The attractions of Oldhampton have evidently proved too strong for her," he said a little drily. "If she had come by the afternoon train, she would have been here an hour ago."

Sara looked troubled.

"Oh, but she **must** be here--somewhere," she insisted rather anxiously.

"Shall I see if I can find her for you?" suggested Trent stiffly.

Sara, sensing his wish to be gone and genuinely disturbed at Molly's non-appearance, acquiesced.

"I should be very glad if you would," she answered. Then turning to Miles, she went on: "I can't think where she can be. Somehow, Molly has become rather--difficult, lately."

Herrick smiled.

"Don't look so distressed. It is only a little ebullition of *la jeunesse*."

Sara turned to him swiftly.

"Then you've noticed it, too--that she is different?"

He nodded.

"Lookers-on see most of the game, you know. And I'm essentially a looker-on." He bit back a quick sigh, and went on hastily: "But I don't think you need worry about our Molly's vagaries. She's too sound *au fond* to get into real mischief."

"She wouldn't mean to," conceded Sara. "But she is----" She hesitated.

"Youthfully irresponsible," suggested Miles. "Let it go at that."

Sara looked at him affectionately, reflecting that Trent's black cynicism made a striking foil to the serene and constant charity of Herrick's outlook.

"You always look for the best in people, Miles," she said appreciatively.

"I have to. Don't you see, people are my whole world. I'm cut off from everything else. If I didn't look for the best in them, I should want to kill myself. And I'm pretty lucky," he added, smiling humorously. "I generally find what I'm looking for."

At this moment Trent returned with the news that Molly was nowhere to be found. It was evident she had not come to Greenacres at all.

Sara rose, feeling oddly apprehensive.

"Then I think I shall go home and see if she has arrived there yet," she said. She smiled down at Miles. "Even irresponsibility needs checking--if carried too far."

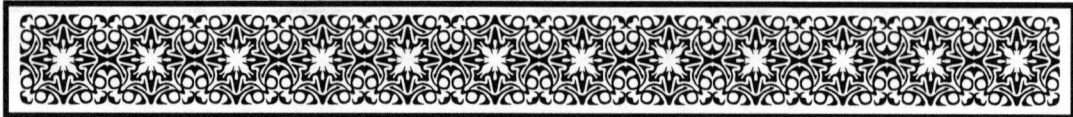

CHAPTER XVI
THE FLIGHT

The first person Sara encountered on her return to Sunnyside was Jane Crab, unmistakably bursting to impart some news.

"The doctor's going away, miss," she announced, flinging her bombshell without preliminary.

"Going away?" Sara's surprise was entirely gratifying, and Jane continued volubly--

"Yes, miss. A telegram came for him early in the afternoon, while he was out on his rounds, asking him to go to a friend who is lying at death's door, as you may say. And please, miss, Dr. Selwyn said he would be glad to see you as soon as you came in."

"Very well, I'll go to him at once. Where is Miss Molly? Has she come back yet?"

"Come and gone again, miss. The doctor asked her to send off a wire for him."

"I see." Sara nodded somewhat abstractly. She was still wondering confusedly why Molly had failed to put in any appearance at Greenacres. "What time did she come in?"

"About a quarter of an hour ago, miss. She missed the early train back from Oldhampton."

Sara's instant feeling of relief was tempered by a mild element of self-reproach. She had been agitating herself about nothing--allowing her uneasiness about Molly to become a perfect obsession, leading her into the wildest imaginings. Here had she been disquieting herself the entire afternoon because Molly had not turned up as arranged, and after all, the simple, commonplace explanation of the matter was that she had missed her train!

Smiling over the groundlessness of her fears, Sara hastened away to Selwyn's study, and found him, seated at his desk, scribbling some hurried motes concerning various cases among his patients for the enlightenment of the medical man who was taking charge of the practice during his absence.

"Oh, there you are, Sara!" he exclaimed, laying down his pen as she entered. "I'm glad you have come back before I go. I'm off in half-an-hour. Did Jane tell you?"

"Yes. I'm very sorry your friend is so ill."

Selwyn's face clouded over.

"I'd like to see him again," he answered simply. "We haven't met for some years--not since my wife's health brought me to Monkshaven--but we were good pals at one time, he and I. Luckily, I've been able to arrange with Dr. Mitchell to include my patients in his round, and if you'll take charge of everything here at home, Sara, I shall have nothing to worry about while I'm away."

"Of course I will. It's very nice of you to entrust your family to my care so confidently."

"Quite confidently," he replied. "I'm not afraid of anything going wrong if you're at the helm."

"How long do you expect to be away?" asked Sara presently.

"A couple of days at the outside. I hope to get back the day after to-morrow."

Denuded of Selwyn's big, kindly presence, the house seemed curiously silent. Even Jane Crab appeared to feel the effect of his absence, and strove less forcefully with her pots and pans--which undoubtedly made for an increase of peace and qui-et--while Molly was frankly depressed, stealing restlessly in and out of the rooms like some haunting shadow.

"What on earth's the matter with you?" Sara asked her laughingly. "Hasn't your father ever been away from home before? You're wandering about like an uneasy spirit!"

"I *am* an uneasy spirit," responded Molly bluntly. "I feel as though I'd a cold coming on, and I always like Dad to doctor me when I'm ill."

"I can doctor a cold," affirmed Sara briskly. "Put your feet in hot water and mustard to-night and stay in bed to-morrow."

Molly considered the proposed remedies in silence.

"Perhaps I *will* stay in bed to-morrow," she said, at last, reluctantly. "Should you mind? We were going down to see the Lavender Lady, you remember."

"I'll go alone. Anyway"--smiling--"if you're safely tucked up in bed, I shall know you're not getting into any mischief while Doctor Dick's away! But very likely the hot water and mustard will put you all right."

"Perhaps it will," agreed Molly hopefully.

The next morning, however, found her in bed, snuffling and complaining of headache, and pathetically resigned to the idea of spending the day between the sheets. Obviously she was in no fit state to inflict her company on other people, so, in the afternoon, after settling her comfortably with a new novel and a box of cigarettes at her bedside, Sara took her solitary way to Rose Cottage.

There she found Garth Trent, sitting beside Herrick's couch and deep in an enthusiastic discussion of amateur photography. But, immediately on her entrance, the eager, interested expression died out of his face, and very shortly after tea he made his farewells, nor could any soft blandishments on the part of the Lavender Lady prevail upon him to remain longer.

Sara felt hurt and resentful. Since the day of the expedition to Devil's Hood Island, Trent had punctiliously avoided being in her company whenever circumstances would permit him to do so, and she was perfectly aware that it was her presence at Rose Cottage which was responsible for his early departure this afternoon.

A gleam of anger flickered in the black depths of her eyes as he shook hands.

"I'm sorry I've driven you away," she flashed at him beneath her breath, with a bitterness akin to his own. He made no answer, merely releasing her hand rather quickly, as though something in her words had flicked him on the raw.

"What a pity Mr. Trent had to leave so soon," remarked Miss Lavinia, with innocent regret, when he had gone. "I'm afraid we shall never persuade him to be really sociable, poor dear man! He seems a little moody to-day, don't you think?"-- hesitating delicately.

"He's a bore!" burst out Sara succinctly.

Miles shook his head.

"No, I don't think that," he said. "But he's a very sick man. In my opinion, Trent's had his soul badly mauled at some time or other."

"He needn't advertise the fact, then," retorted Sara, unappeased. "We all get our share of ill-luck. Garth behaves as if he had the monopoly."

"There are some scars which can't be hidden," replied Miles quietly.

Sara smiled a little. There was never any evading Herrick's broad tolerance of human nature.

It was nearly an hour later when at last she took her way homewards, carrying in her heart, in spite of herself, something of the gentle serenity that seemed to be a part of the very atmosphere at Rose Cottage.

Outside, the calm and fragrance of a June evening awaited her. Little, delicate, sweet-smelling airs floated over the tops of the hedges from the fields beyond, and now and then a few stray notes of a blackbird's song stole out from a plantation near at hand, breaking off suddenly and dying down into drowsy, contented little cluckings and twitterings.

Across the bay the sun was dipping towards the horizon, flinging along the face of the waters great shafts of lambent gold and orange, that split into a thousand particles of shimmering light as the ripples caught them up and played with them, and finally tossed them back again to the sun from the shining curve of a wave's sleek side.

It was all very tranquil and pleasant, and Sara strolled leisurely along, soothed into a half-waking dream by the peaceful influences of the moment. Even the manifold perplexities and tangles of life seemed to recede and diminish in importance at the touch of old Mother Nature's comforting hand. After all, there was much, very much, that was beautiful and pleasant still left to enjoy.

It is generally at moments like these, when we are sinking into a placid quiescence of endurance, that Fate sees fit to prod us into a more active frame of mind.

In this particular instance destiny manifested itself in the unassuming form of Black Brady, who slid suddenly down from the roadside hedge, amid a crackling of branches and rattle of rubble, and appeared in front of Sara's astonished eyes just as she was nearing home.

"Beg pardon, miss"--Brady tugged at a forelock of curly black hair--"I was just on me way to your place."

"To Sunnyside? Why, is Mrs. Brady ill again?" asked Sara kindly.

"No, miss, thank you, she's doing nicely." He paused a moment as though at a loss how to continue. Then he burst out: "It's about Miss Molly--the doctor bein' away and all."

"About Miss Molly?" Sara felt a sudden clutch at her heart. "What do you mean? Quick, Brady, what is it?"

"Well, miss, I've just seed 'er go off 'long o' Mr. Kent in his big motor-car. They took the London road, and"--here Brady shuffled his feet with much embarrassment--"seein' as Mr. Kent's a married man, I'll be bound he's up to no good wi' Miss Molly."

Sara could have stamped with vexation. The little fool--oh! The utter little *fool*--to go off joy-riding in an evening like that! A break-down of any kind, with a consequent delay in returning, and all Monkshaven would be buzzing with the tale!

For the moment, however, there was nothing to be done except to put Black Brady in his place and pray for Molly's speedy return.

"Well, Brady," she said coldly, "I imagine Mr. Kent's a good enough driver to bring Miss Selwyn back safely. I don't think there's anything to worry about."

Brady stared at her out of his sullen eyes.

"You haven't understood, miss," he said doggedly. "Mr. Kent isn't for bringing Miss Molly back again. They'd their luggage along wi' 'em in the car, and Mr. Kent, he stopped at the 'Cliff' to have the tank filled up and took a matter of another half-dozen cans o' petrol with 'im."

In an instant the whole dreadful significance of the thing leaped into Sara's mind. Molly had bolted--run away with Lester Kent!

It was easy enough now, in the flashlight kindled by Brady's slow, inexorable summing up of detail, to see the drift of recent happenings, the meaning of each small, disconcerting fact that added a fresh link to the chain of probability.

Molly's unwonted secretiveness; her strange, uncertain moods; her embarrassment at finding she was expected at Greenacres when she had presumably agreed to meet Lester Kent in Oldhampton; and, last of all, the sudden "cold" which had developed coincidentally with her father's absence from home and which had secured her freedom from any kind of supervision for the afternoon. And the opportunity of clinching arrangements--probably already planned and dependent only on a convenient moment--had been provided by her errand to the post office to send off her father's telegram--it being as easy to send two telegrams as one.

The colour ebbed slowly from Sara's face as full realization dawned upon her, and she swayed a little where she stood. With rough kindliness Brady stretched out a grimy hand and steadied her.

"'Ere, don't' take on, miss. They won't get very far. I didn't, so to speak, *fill* the petrol tank"--with a grin--"and there ain't more than two o' they cans I slipped aboard the car as 'olds more'n air. The rest was empties"--the grin widened enjoy-ably--"which I shoved in well to the back. Mr. Kent won't travel eighty miles afore 'e calls a 'alt, I reckon."

Sara looked at Brady's cunning, kindly face almost with affection.

"Why did you do that?" she asked swiftly.

"I've owed Mr. Lester Kent summat these three years," he answered compla-cently. "And I never forgets to pay back. I owed you summat, too, Miss Tennant. I haven't forgot how you spoke up for me when I was catched poachin'."

Sara held out her hand to him impulsively, and Brady sheepishly extended his own grubby paw to meet it.

"You've more than paid me back, Brady," she said warmly. "Thank you."

Turning away, she hurried up the road, leaving Brady staring alternately at his right hand and at her receding figure.

"She's rare gentry, is Miss Tennant," he remarked with conviction, and then slouched off to drink himself blind at "The Jolly Sailorman." Black Brady was, after all, only an inexplicable bundle of good and bad impulses--very much like his bet-ters.

Arrived at the house, Sara fled breathlessly upstairs to Molly's room. Jane Crab was standing in the middle of it, staring dazedly at all the evidences of a hasty de-parture which surrounded her--an overturned chair here, an empty hat-box there, drawers pulled out, and clothes tossed heedlessly about in every direction. In her hand she held a chemist's parcel, neatly sealed and labeled; she was twisting it round and round in her trembling, gnarled old fingers.

At the sound of Sara's entrance, she turned with an exclamation of relief.

"Oh, Miss Sara! I'm main glad you've come! Whatever's happened? Miss Molly was here in bed not three parts of an hour ago!" Then, her boot-button eyes still roving round the room, she made a sudden dart towards the dressing-table. "Here, miss, 'tis a note she's left for you!" she exclaimed, snatching it up and thrusting it into Sara's hands.

Written in Molly's big, sprawling, childish hand, the note was a pathetic mixture of confession and apology--

"I feel a perfect pig, Sara mine, leaving you behind to face Father, but it was my only chance of getting away, as I know Dad would have refused to let me marry for years and years. He never *will* realize that I'm grown-up. And Lester and I couldn't wait all that time.

"I felt an awful fraud last night, letting you fuss over my supposed 'cold,' you dear thing. Do forgive me. And you must come and stay with us the minute we get back from our honeymoon. We are to be married to-morrow morning. "--MOLLY.

"P.S.--Don't worry--it's all quite proper and respectable. I'm to go straight to the house of one of Lester's sisters in London.

"P.P.S.--I'm frantically happy."

Sara's eyes were wet when she finished the perusal of the hastily scribbled letter. "We are to be married to-morrow morning!" The blind, pathetic confidence of it! And if Black Brady had spoken the truth, if Lester Kent were already a married man, to-morrow morning would convert the trusting, wayward baby of a woman, with her adorable inconsistencies and her big, generous heart, into something Sara dared not contemplate. The thought of the look in those brown-gold eyes, when Molly should know the truth, brought a lump into her throat.

She turned to Jane Crab.

"Listen to me, Jane," she said tersely. "Miss Molly's run away with Mr. Lester Kent. She thinks he's going to marry her. But he can't--he's married already----"

"Sakes alive!" Just that one brief exclamation, and then suddenly Jane's lower lip began to work convulsively, and two tears squeezed themselves out of her little eyes, and her whole face puckered up like a baby's.

Sara caught her by the arm and shook her.

"Don't cry!" she said vehemently. "You haven't time! We've got to save her-- we've got to get her back before any one knows. Do you understand? Stop crying at once!"

Jane reacted promptly to the fierce imperative, and sniffingly choked back her tears. Suddenly her eyes fell on the little package from the chemist which she still held clutched in her hand.

"The artfulness of her!" she ejaculated indignantly. "Asking me to go along to the chemist's and bring her back some aspirin for her headache! And me, like a fool, suspecting nothing, off I goes! There's the stuff!"--viciously flinging the chemist's parcel on to the floor. "Eh! Miss Molly'll have more than a headache to face, I'm thinking!"

"But she *mustn't*, Jane! We've got to get her back, somehow."

Though Sara spoke with such assured conviction, she was inwardly racked with anxiety. What *could* they do--two forlorn women? And to whom could they turn for help? Miles? He was lame. He was no abler to help than they themselves. And Selwyn was away, out of reach!

"We must get her back," she repeated doggedly.

"And how, may I ask, Miss Sara?" inquired Jane bitterly. "Be you goin' to run after the motor-car, mayhap?"

For a moment Sara was silent. The sarcastic query had set the spark to the tinder, and now she was thinking rapidly, some semblance of a plan emerging at last from the chaotic turmoil of her mind.

Garth Trent! He could help her! He had a car--Sara did not know its pace, but she was certain Trent could be trusted to get every ounce out of it that was possible. Between them--he and she--they would bring Molly back to safety!

She turned swiftly to Jane Crab.

"Come to the stable and help me put in the Doctor's pony, Jane. You know how, don't you?"

"Yes, miss, I've helped the master many a time. But you ain't going to catch no motor with old Toby, Miss Sara."

"No, I don't expect to. I'm gong to drive across to Far End. Mr. Trent will help us. Don't worry, Jane"--as the two made their way to the stable and Jane strangled a sob--"we'll bring Miss Molly back. And, listen! Mrs. Selwyn isn't to hear a word of this. Do you understand? If she asks you anything, tell her that Miss Molly and I are dining out. That'll be true enough, too," added Sara grimly, "if we dine at all!"

Jane sniffed, and swallowed loudly.

"Yes, miss," she said submissively. "You and Miss Molly are dining out. I won't forget."

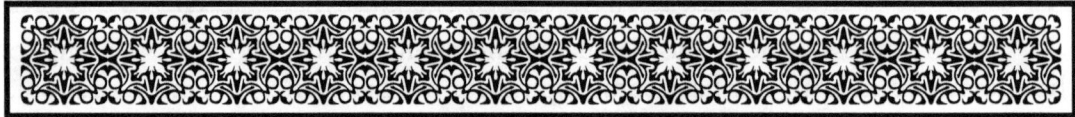

CHAPTER XVII
THEY WHO PURSUED

Selwyn's pony had rarely before found himself hustled along at the pace at which Sara drove him. She let him take his time up the hills, knowing, as every good horse-woman knows, that if you press your horse against the hill, he will only flag the sooner and that you will lose more than you gain. But down the hills and along the flat, Sara, with hands and whip, kept Toby going at an amazing pace. Perhaps something of her own urgency communicated itself to the good-hearted beast, for he certainly made a great effort and brought her to Far End in a shorter time than she had deemed possible.

Exactly as she pulled him to a standstill, the front door opened and Garth himself appeared. He had heard the unwonted sound of wheels on the drive, and now, as he recognized his late visitor, an expression of extreme surprise crossed his face.

"Miss Tennant!" he exclaimed in astonished tones.

"Yes. Can your man take my pony? And, please may I come in? I--I must see you alone for a few minutes."

Trent glanced at her searchingly as his ear caught the note of strain in her voice.

Summoning Judson to take charge of the pony and trap, he led the way into the comfortable, old fashioned hall and wheeled forward an armchair.

"Sit down," he said composedly. "Now"--as she obeyed--"tell me what is the matter."

His manner held a quiet friendliness. The chill indifference he had accorded her of late--even earlier that same day at Rose Cottage--had vanished, and his curiously bright eyes regarded her with sympathetic interest.

To the man as he appeared at the moment, it was no difficult matter for Sara to unburden her heart, and a few minutes later he was in possession of all the facts concerning Molly's flight.

"I don't know whether Mr. Kent is really a married man or not," she added in conclusion. "Brady declares that he is."

"He is," replied Trent curtly. "Very much married. His first wife divorced him, and, since then, he has married again."

"Oh----!" Sara half-rose from her seat, her face blanching. Not till that moment did she realize how much in her inmost heart she had been relying on the hope that Garth might be able to contradict Black Brady's statement.

"Don't worry." Garth laid his hands on her shoulders and pushed her gently back into her chair again. "Don't worry. Thanks to Brady's stroke of genius about the petrol--I've evidently underestimated the man's good points--I think I can promise you that you shall have Miss Molly safely back at Sunnyside in the course of a few hours. That is, if you are willing to trust me in the matter."

"Of course I will trust you," she answered simply. Somehow it seemed as though a great burden had been lifted from her shoulders since she had confided her trouble to Garth.

"Thank you," he said quietly. "Now, while Judson gets the car round, you must have a glass of wine."

"No--oh, no!"--hastily--"I don't want anything."

"Allow me to know better than you do in this case," he replied, smiling.

He left the room, presently returning with a bottle of champagne and a couple of glasses.

"Oh, please--I'd so much rather start at once," she protested. "I really don't want anything. Do let us hurry!"

"I'm sorry, but I've no intention of starting until you have drunk this"--filling and handing one of the glasses to her.

Rather than waste time in further argument, she accepted it, only to find that her hand was shaking uncontrollably, so that the edge of the glass chattered against her teeth.

"I--I can't!" she gasped helplessly. Now that she had shared her burden of responsibility, the demands of the last half-hour's anxiety and strain were making themselves felt.

With a swift movement Garth took the glass from her, and, supporting her with his other arm, held it to her lips.

"Drink it down," he said authoritatively. Then, as she paused: "All of it!"

In a few minutes the wine had brought the colour back to her face, and she felt more like herself again.

"I'm all right, now," she said. "I'm sorry I was such a fool. But--but this business about Molly has given me rather a shock, I suppose."

"Naturally. Now, if you're ready, we'll make a start."

She rose, and he surveyed her slight figure in its thin muslin gown with some amusement.

"Not quite a suitable costume for motoring by night," he remarked. He picked up one of the two big fur coats Mrs. Judson had brought into the room. "Here, put this on." Then, when he had fastened it round her and turned the collar up about her neck, he stood looking at her for a moment in silence.

The whole of her slender form was hidden beneath the voluminous folds of the big coat, which had been originally designed to fit Garth's own proportions, and against the high fur collar her delicate cameo face, with its white skin and scarlet lips and its sombre, night-black eyes, emerged like some vivid flower from its sheath.

Trent laughed shortly.

"Beauty--in the garment of the Beast," he commented. Then, briskly: "Come along. Judson will have the car ready by now."

Sara stepped into the car and he tucked the rugs carefully round her. Then, directing Judson to drive the Selwyn pony and trap back to Sunnyside, he took his place at the wheel and the car slid noiselessly away down the broad drive.

"The surprising discovery of the doctor's pony and trap at Far End to-morrow morning would require explanation," he observed grimly to Sara. She blessed his thoughtfulness.

"What about Judson?" she asked. "Is he reliable? Or do you think he will--talk?"

"Judson," replied Garth, "has been in my service long enough to know the meaning of the word 'discretion.'"

Trent drove the car steadily enough through town, but, as soon as they emerged on to the great London main road, he let her out and they swept rapidly along through the lingering summer twilight.

"Are you nervous?" he asked. "Do you mind forty or fifty miles an hour when we've a clear stretch ahead of us?"

"Eighty, if you like," she replied succinctly.

She felt the car leap forward like a living thing beneath them as it gathered speed.

"Do you think--is it possible that we can overtake them?" she asked anxiously.

"It's got to be done," he answered, and she was conscious of the quiet driving-force that lay behind the speech--the stubborn resolution of the man which she had begun to recognize as his most dominant characteristic.

She wondered, as she had so often wondered before, whether any one had ever yet succeeded in turning Garth Trent aside from his set purpose, whatever it might chance to be. She could not imagine his yielding to either threats or persuasions. However much it might cost him, he would carry out his intention to the bitter end, even though its fulfillment might involve the shattering of the whole significance of life.

"Besides,"--his voice cut across the familiar tenor of her thoughts--"Kent will probably stop to dine at some hotel *en route*. We shan't. We'll feed as we go."

"Oh--h!" A gasp of horrified recollection escaped her. "I never thought of it! Of course you've had no dinner!"

He laughed. "Have you?" he asked amusedly.

"No, but that's different."

"Well, we'll even matters up by having some sandwiches together presently. Mrs. Judson has packed some in."

Sara was silent, inwardly dwelling on the fact that no least detail ever seemed to escape Garth's attention. Even in the hurry of their departure, and with the whole scheme of Molly's rescue to envisage, he had yet found time to order due provision for the journey.

An hour later they pulled up at the principal hotel of the first big town on the route, and Garth elicited the fact that a car answering to the description of Lester Kent's had stopped there, but only for a bare ten minutes which had enabled its occupants to snatch a hasty meal.

"They've been here and gone straight on," he reported to Sara. "Evidently

Kent's taking no chances"--grimly. And a moment later they were on their way once more. Dusk deepened into dark, and the car's great headlights cut out a blazing track of gold in front of them as they rushed along the pale ribbon of road that stretched ahead--mile after interminable mile.

On either side, dark woods merged into the deeper darkness of the encroaching night, seeming to slip past them like some ghostly marching army as the car tore its way between the ranks of shadowy trunks. Overhead, a few stars crept out, puncturing the expanse of darkening sky--pale, tremulous sparks of light in contrast with the steady, warmly golden glow that streamed from the lights of the car.

Presently Garth slackened speed.

"Why are you stopping?" Sara's voice, shrilling a little with anxiety, came to him out of the darkness.

"I'm not stopping. I'm only slowing down a bit, because I think it's quite feeding time. Do you mind opening those two leather attachments fixed in front of you? Such nectar and ambrosia as Mrs. Judson has provided is in there."

Sara leaned forward, and unbuckling the lid of a flattish leather case which, together with another containing a flask, was slung just opposite her, withdrew from within it a silver sandwich-box. She snapped open the lid and proffered the box to Garth.

"Help yourself. And--do you mind"--he spoke a little uncertainly and the darkness hid the expression of his face from her--"handing me my share--in pieces suitable for human consumption? This is a bad bit of road, and I want both hands for driving the car."

In silence Sara broke the sandwiches and fed him, piece by piece, while he bent over the wheel, driving steadily onward.

The little, intimate action sent a curious thrill through her. It seemed in some way to draw them together, effacing the memory of those weeks of bitter indifference which lay behind them. Such a thing would have been grotesquely impossible of performance in the atmosphere of studied formality supplied by their estrangement, and Sara smiled a little to herself under cover of the darkness.

"One more mouthful!" she announced as she halved the last sandwich.

An instant later she felt his lips brush her fingers in a sudden, burning kiss, and she withdrew her hand as though stung.

She was tingling from head to foot, every nerve of her a-thrill, and for a moment she felt as though she hated him. He had been so kind, so friendly, so essentially the good comrade in this crisis occasioned by Molly's flight, and now he had spoilt it all--playing the lover once more when he had shown her clearly that he meant nothing by it.

Apparently he sensed her attitude--the quick withdrawal of spirit which had accompanied the more physical retreat.

"Forgive me!" he said, rather low. "I won't offend again."

She made no answer, and presently she felt the car sliding slowly to a standstill. A sudden panic assailed her.

"What is it? What are you doing?" she asked, quick fear in her sharply spoken question.

He laughed shortly.

"You needn't be afraid--" he began.

"I'm not!" she interpolated hastily.

"Excuse me," he said drily, "but you are. You don't trust me in the slightest degree. Well"--she could guess, rather than see, the shrug which accompanied the words--"I can't blame you. It's my own fault, I suppose."

He braked the car, and she quivered to a dead stop, throbbing like a live thing in the darkness.

"You must forgive me for being so material," he went on composedly, "but I want a drink, and I'm not acrobat enough to manage that, even with your help, while we're doing thirty miles an hour."

He lifted out the flask, and, when they had both drunk, Sara meekly took it from him and proceeded to adjust the screw cap and fit the silver cup back into its place over the lower half of the flask.

Simultaneously she felt the car begin to move forward, and then, quite how it happened she never knew, but, fumbling in the darkness, she contrived to knock the cup sharply against the flask, and it flew out of her hand and over the side of the car. Impulsively she leaned out, trying to snatch it back as it fell, and, in the same instant, something seemed to give way, and she felt herself hurled forward into space. The earth rushed up to meet her, a sound as of many waters roared in her ears, and then the blank darkness of unconsciousness swallowed her up.

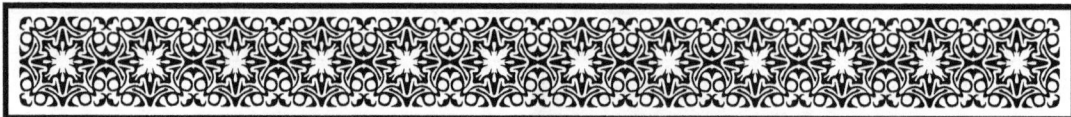

CHAPTER XVIII
THE REVELATION OF THE NIGHT

Thank God, she's only stunned!"

The words, percolating slowly through the thick, blankety mist that seemed to have closed about her, impressed themselves on Sara's mind with a vague, confused suggestion of their pertinence. It was as though some one--she wasn't quite sure who--had suddenly given voice to her own immediate sensation of relief.

At first she could not imagine for what reason she should feel so specially grateful and relieved. Gradually, however, the mists began to clear away and recollection of a kind returned to her.

She remembered dropping something--she couldn't recall precisely what it was that she had dropped, but she knew she had made a wild clutch at it and tried to save it as it fell. Then--she was remembering more distinctly now--something against which she had been leaning--she couldn't recall what that was, either--gave way suddenly, and for the fraction of a second she had known she was going to fall and be killed, or, at the least, horribly hurt and mutilated.

And now, it seemed, she had not been hurt at all! She was in no pain; only her head felt unaccountably heavy. But for that, she was really very comfortable. Some one was holding her--it was almost like lying back in a chair--and against her cheek she could feel the soft warmth of fur.

"Sara--beloved!"

It was Garth's voice, quite close to her ear. He was holding her in his arms.

Ah! She knew now! They were on the island together, and he had just asked her if she cared. Of course she cared! It was sheer happiness to lie in his arms, with closed eyes, and hear his voice--that deep, unhappy voice of his--grow suddenly so incredibly soft and tender.

"You're mine, now, sweet! Mine to hold just for this once, dear of my heart!"

No, that couldn't be right, after all, because it wasn't Garth who loved her. He had only pretended to care for her by way of amusing himself. It must be Tim who was talking to her--Tim, whom she was going to marry.

Then, suddenly, the mists cleared quite away, and Sara came back to full consciousness and to the knowledge of where she was and of what had happened.

Her first instinct, to open her eyes and speak, was checked by a swift, unexpected movement on the part of Garth. All at once, he had gathered her up into his arms, and, holding her face pressed close against his own, was pouring into her ears a torrent of burning, passionate words of love--love triumphant, worshipping, agonizing, and last of all, brokenly, desperately abandoning all right or claim.

"And I've got to live without you . . . die without you . . . My God, it's hard!"

In the darkness and solitude of the night--as he believed, alone with the unconscious form of the woman he loved in his arms--Garth bared his very soul. There was nothing hidden any longer, and Sara knew at last that even as she herself loved, so was she loved again.

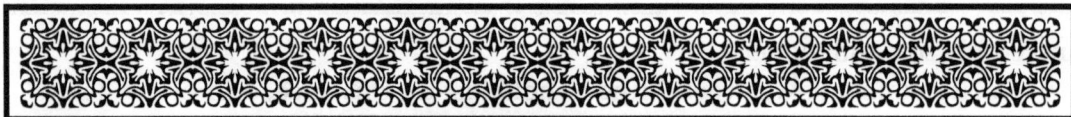

CHAPTER XIX
THE JOURNEY'S END

Sara stirred a little and opened her eyes. Deep within herself she was ashamed of those brief moments of assumed unconsciousness--those moments which had shown her a strong man's soul stripped naked of all pride and subterfuge--his heart and soul as he alone knew them.

But, none the less, she felt gloriously happy. Nothing could ever hurt her badly again. Garth loved her!

Since, for some reason, he himself would never have drawn aside the veil and let her know the truth, she was glad--glad that she had peered unbidden through the rent which the stress of the moment had torn in his iron self-command and reticence. Just as she had revealed herself to him on the island, in a moment of equal strain, so he had now revealed himself to her, and they were quits.

"I'm all right," she announced, struggling into a sitting position. "I'm not hurt."

"Sit still a minute, while I fetch you some brandy from the car." Garth spoke in a curiously controlled voice.

He was back again in a moment, and the raw spirit made her catch her breath as it trickled down her throat.

"Thank God we had only just begun to move," he said. "Otherwise you must have been half-killed."

"What happened?" she asked curiously. "How did I fall out?"

"The door came open. That damned fool, Judson, didn't shut it properly. Are you sure you're not hurt?"

"Quite sure. My head aches rather."

"That's very probable. You were stunned for a minute or two."

Suddenly the recollection of their errand returned to her.

"Molly! Good Heavens, how much time have we wasted? How long has this silly business taken?" she demanded, in a frenzy of apprehension.

Garth surveyed her oddly in the glow of one of the car's side-lights, which he had carried back with him when he fetched the brandy.

"Five minutes, I should think," he said, adding under his breath: "Or half eternity!"

"Five minutes! Is that all? Then do let's hurry on."

She took a few steps in the direction of the car, then stopped and wavered. She felt curiously shaky, and her legs seemed as though they did not belong to her.

In a moment Garth was at her side, and had lifted her up in his arms. He carried her swiftly across the few yards that intervened between them and the car, and settled her gently into her seat.

"Do you feel fit to go on?" he asked.

"Of course I do. We must--bring Molly back." Even her voice refused to obey the dictates of her brain, and quavered weakly.

"Well, try to rest a little. Don't talk, and perhaps you'll go to sleep."

He restarted the car, and, taking his seat once more at the wheel, drove on at a smooth and easy pace.

Sara leaned back in silence at his side, conscious of a feeling of utter lassitude. In spite of her anxiety about Molly, a curious contentment had stolen over her. The long strain of the past weeks had ended--ended in the knowledge that Garth loved her, and nothing else seemed to matter very much. Moreover, she was physically exhausted. Her fall had shaken her badly, and she wanted nothing better than to lie back quietly against the padded cushions of the car, lulled by the rhythmic throb of the engine, and glide on through the night indefinitely, knowing that Garth was there, close to her, all the time.

Presently her quiet, even breathing told that she slept, and Garth, stooping over her to make sure, accelerated the speed, and soon the car shot forward through the darkness at a pace which none but a driver very certain of his skill would have dared to attempt.

When, an hour later, Sara awoke, she felt amazingly refreshed. Only a slight headache remained to remind her of her recent accident.

"Where are we?" she asked eagerly. "How long have I been asleep?"

"Feeling better?" queried Garth, reassured by the stronger note in her voice.

"Quite all right, thanks. But tell me where we are?"

"Nearly at our journey's end, I take it," he replied grimly, suddenly slackening speed. "There's a stationary car ahead there on the left, do you see? That will be our friends, I expect, held up by petrol shortage, thanks to Jim Brady."

Sara peered ahead, and on the edge of the broad ribbon of light that stretched in front of them she could discern a big car, drawn up to one side of the road, its headlights shut off, its side-lights glimmering warningly against its dark bulk.

Exactly as they drew level with it, Garth pulled up to a standstill. Then a muttered curse escaped him, and simultaneously Sara gave vent to an exclamation of dismay. The car was empty.

Garth sprang out and flashed a lamp over the derelict.

"Yes," he said, "that's Kent's car right enough."

Sara's heart sank.

"What can have become of them?" she exclaimed. She glanced round her as though she half suspected that Kent and Molly might be hiding by the roadside.

Meanwhile Garth had peered into the tank and was examining the petrol cans stowed away in the back of the deserted car.

"Run dry!" he announced, coming back to his own car. "That's what has happened."

"And what can we do now?" asked Sara despondently.

He laughed a little.

"Faint heart!" he chided. "What can we do now? Why, ask ourselves what Kent would naturally have done when he found himself landed high and dry?"

"I don't know what he *could* do--in the middle of nowhere?" she answered doubtfully.

"Only we don't happen to be in the middle of nowhere! We're just about a couple of miles from a market town where abides a nice little inn whence petrol can be obtained. Kent and Miss Molly have doubtless trudged there on foot, and wakened up mine host, and they'll hire a trap and drive back with a fresh supply of oil. By Jove!"--with a grim laugh--"How Kent must have cursed when he discovered the trick Brady played on him!"

Ten minutes later, leaving their car outside, Garth and Sara walked boldly up to the inn of which he had spoken. The door stood open, and a light was burning in the coffee-room. Evidently some one had just arrived.

Garth glanced into the room, then, standing back, he motioned Sara to enter.

Sara stepped quickly over the threshold and then paused, swept by an infinite compassion and tenderness almost maternal in its solicitude.

Molly was sitting hunched up in a chair, her face half hidden against her arm, every drooping line of her slight young figure bespeaking weariness. She had taken off her hat and tossed it on to the table, and now she had dropped into a brief, uneasy slumber born of sheer fatigue and excitement.

"Molly!"

At the sound of Sara's voice she opened big, startled eyes and stared incredulously.

Sara moved swiftly to her.

"Molly dear," she said, "I've come to take you home."

At that Molly started up, broad awake in an instant.

"You? How did you come here?" she stammered. Then, realization waking in her eyes: "But I'm not coming back with you. We've only stopped for petrol. Lester's outside, somewhere, seeing about it now. We're driving back to the car."

"Yes, I know. But you're not going on with Mr. Kent"--very gently--"you're coming home with us."

Molly drew herself up, flaring passionate young defiance, talking glibly of love, and marriage, and living her own life--all the beautiful, romantic nonsense that comes so readily to the soft lips of youth, the beckoning rose and gold of sunrise--and of mirage--which is all youth's untrained eyes can see.

Sara was getting desperate. The time was flying. At any moment Kent might return. Garth signaled to her from the doorway.

"You must tell her," he said gruffly. "If Kent returns before we go, we shall have a scene. Get her away quick."

Sara nodded. Then she came back to Molly's side.

"My dear," she said pitifully. "You can never marry Lester Kent, because--because he has a wife already."

"I don't believe it!" The swift denial leaped from Molly's lips.

But she did believe it, nevertheless. No one who knew Sara could have looked into her eyes at that moment and doubted that she was speaking not only what she believed to be, but what she *knew* to be, the ugly truth.

Suddenly Molly crumpled up. As, between them, Garth and Sara hurried her away to the car, there was no longer anything of the regal young goddess about her. She was just a child--a tired, frightened child whose eyes had been suddenly opened to the quicksands whereon her feet were set, and, like a child, she turned instinctively and clung to the dear, familiar people from home, who were mercifully at hand to shield her when her whole world had suddenly grown new and strange and very terrible. . . .

On, on through the night roared the big car, with Garth bending low over the wheel in front, while, in the back-seat Molly huddled forlornly into the curve of Sara's arm.

A few questions had elicited the whole foolish story of Lester Kent's infatuation, and of the steps he had taken to enmesh poor simple-hearted Molly in the toils--first, by lending her money, then, when he found that the loan had scared her, by buying her pictures and surrounding her with an atmosphere of adulation which momentarily blinded her from forming any genuine estimate either of the value of his criticism or of the sincerity of his desire to purchase.

Once the head resting against Sara's shoulder was lifted, and a wistfully incredulous voice asked, very low--

"You are sure he is married, Sara,--*quite sure*?"

"Quite sure, Molly," came the answer.

And later, as they were nearing home, Molly's hardly-bought philosophy of life revealed itself in the brief comment: "It's very easy to make a fool of oneself."

"Probably Mr. Kent has found that out--by this time," replied Sara with a grim flash of humour.

A faint, involuntary chuckle in response premised that ultimately Molly might be able to take a less despondent view of the night's proceedings.

It was between two and three in the morning when at length the travelers climbed stiffly out of the car at the gateway of Sunnyside and made their way up the little tiled path that led to the front door. The latter opened noiselessly at their approach and Jane, who had evidently been watching for them, stood on the threshold.

Her small, beady eyes were red-rimmed with sleeplessness--and with the slow, difficult tears that now and again had overflowed as hour after hour crawled by, bringing no sign of the wanderers' return--and the shadows of fatigue that had hollowed her weather-beaten cheeks wrung a sympathetic pang from Sara's heart as she realized what those long, inactive hours of helpless anxiety must have meant to the faithful soul.

Jane's glance flew to the drooping, willowy figure clinging to Garth's arm.

"My lamb! . . . Oh! Miss Molly dear, they've brought 'ee back!" Impulsively she caught hold of Garth's coat-sleeve. "Thank God you've brought them back, sir, and now there's none as need ever know aught but that they've been in their beds all the blessed night!" Her lips were shaking, drawn down at the corners like those of a distressed child, but her harsh old voice quivered triumphantly.

A very kindly gleam showed itself in Garth's dark face as he patted the rough, red hand that clutched his coat-sleeve.

"Yes, I've brought them back safely," he said. "Put them to bed, Jane. Miss Sara's fallen out of the car and Miss Molly has tumbled out of heaven, so they're both feeling pretty sore."

But Sara's soreness was far the easier to bear, since it was purely physical. As she lay in bed, at last, utterly weary and exhausted, the recollection of all the horror and anxiety that had followed upon the discovery of Molly's flight fell away from her, and she was only conscious that had it not been for that wild night-ride which Molly's danger had compelled, she would never have known that Garth loved her.

So, out of evil, had come good; out of black darkness had been born the exquisite clear shining of the dawn.

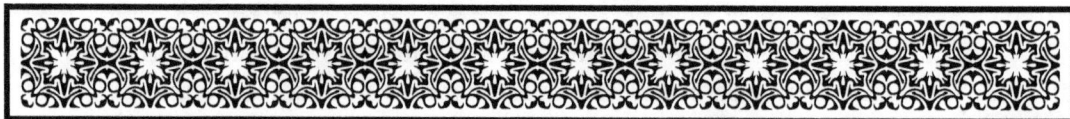

CHAPTER XX
THE SECOND BEST

Sara laid down her pen and very soberly re-read the letter she had just written. It was to Tim Durward, telling him the engagement between them must be at an end, and its accomplishment had been a matter of sore embarrassment and mental struggle. Sara hated giving pain, and she knew that this letter, taking from Tim all--and it was so painfully little--that she had ever given him, must bring very bitter pain to the man to whom, as friend and comrade, she was deeply attached.

It was barely a month since she had promised to marry him, and it was a difficult, ungracious task, and very open to misapprehension, to write and rescind that promise.

Yet it was characteristic of Sara that no other alternative presented itself to her. Now that she was sure Garth cared for her--whether their mutual love must remain for ever unfulfilled, unconsummated, or not--she knew that she could never give herself to any other man.

She folded and sealed the letter, and then sat quietly contemplating the consequences that it might entail. Almost inevitably it would mean a complete estrangement from the Durwards. Elisabeth would be very unlikely ever to forgive her for her treatment of Tim; even kindly hearted Major Durward could not but feel sore about it; and since Garth had not asked her to marry him--and showed no disposition to do any such thing--they would almost certainly fail to understand or sympathize with her point of view.

Sara sighed as she dropped her missive into the letter-box. It meant an end to the pleasant and delightful friendship which had come into her life just at the time when Patrick Lovell's death had left it very empty and desolate.

Two days of suspense ensued while she restlessly awaited Tim's reply. Then, on the third day, he came himself, his eyes incredulous, his face showing traces of the white night her letter had cost him.

He was very gentle with her. There was no bitterness or upbraiding, and he suffered her explanation with a grave patience that hurt her more than any reproaches he could have uttered.

"I believed it was only I who cared, Tim," she told him. "And so I felt free to give you what you wanted--to be your wife, if you cared to take me, knowing I had no love to give. I thought"--she faltered a little--"that I might as well make *some-one* happy! But now that I know he loves me as I love him, I couldn't marry any one else, could I?"

"And are you going to marry him--this man you love?"

"I don't know. He has not asked me to marry him."

"Perhaps he is married already?"

Sara met his eyes frankly.

"I don't know even that."

Tim made a fierce gesture of impatience.

"Is it playing fair--to keep you in ignorance like that?" he demanded.

Sara laughed suddenly.

"Perhaps not. But somehow I don't mind. I am sure he must have a good reason--or else"--with a flash of humour--"some silly man's reason that won't be any obstacle at all!"

"Supposing"--Tim bent over her, his face rather white--"supposing you find--later on--that there is some real obstacle--that he can't marry you, would you come to me--then, Sara?"

She shook her head.

"No, Tim, not now. Don't you see, now that I know he cares for me--everything is altered. I'm not free, now. In a way, I belong to him. Oh! How can I explain? Even though we may never marry, there is a faithfulness of the spirit, Tim. It's--it's the biggest part of love, really----"

She broke off, and presently she felt Tim's hands on her shoulders.

"I think I understand, dear," he said gently. "It's just what I should expect of you. It means the end of everything--everything that matters for me. But--somehow--I would not have you otherwise."

He did not stay very long after that. They talked together a little, promising each other that their friendship should still remain unbroken and unspoilt.

"For," as Tim said, "if I cannot have the best that the world can give--your love, Sara, I need not lose the second best--which is your friendship."

And Sara, watching him from the window as he strode away down the little tiled path, wondered why love comes so often bearing roses in one hand and a sharp goad in the other.

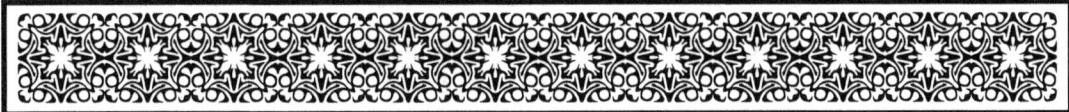

CHAPTER XXI
THE PITILESS ALTAR

Elisabeth was pacing restlessly up and down the broad, flagged terrace at Barrow, impatiently awaiting Tim's return from Monkshaven.

She knew his errand there. He had scarcely needed to tell her the contents of Sara's letter, so swiftly had she summed up the immediate connection between the glimpse she had caught of Sara's handwriting and the shadow on the beloved face.

She moved eagerly to meet him as she heard the soft purr of the motor coming up the drive.

"Well?" she queried, slipping her arm through his and drawing him towards the terrace.

Tim looked at her with troubled eyes. He could guess so exactly what her attitude would be, and he was not going to allow even Elisabeth to say unkind things about the woman he loved. If he could prevent it, she should not think them.

Very gently, and with infinite tact, he told her the result of his interview with Sara, concealing so far as might be his own incalculable hurt.

To his relief, his mother accepted the facts with unexpected tolerance. He could not see her expression, since her eyes veiled themselves with down-dropped lids, but she spoke quite quietly and as though trying to be fair in her judgment. There was no outward sign by which her son might guess the seething torrent of anger and resentment which had been aroused within her.

"But if, as you tell me, Sara doesn't expect to marry this man she cares for, surely she had been unduly hasty? If he can never be anything to her, need she set aside all thought of matrimony?"

Tim stared at his mother in some surprise. There was a superficial worldly wisdom in the speech which he would not have anticipated.

"It seems to me rather absurd," she continued placidly. "Quixotic--the sort of romantic 'live and die unwed' idea that is quite exploded. Girls nowadays don't wither on their virgin stems if the man they want doesn't happen to be in a position to marry them. They marry some one else."

Tim felt almost shocked. From his childhood he had invested his mother with a kind of rarefied grace of mental and moral qualities commensurate with her physical beauty, and her enunciation of the cynical creed of modern times staggered him. It never occurred to him that Elisabeth was probing round in order to extract a clear idea of Sara's attitude in the whole matter, and he forthwith proceeded innocently to give her precisely the information she was seeking.

"Sara isn't like that, mother," he said rather shortly. "It's just the--the crystal purity of her outlook which makes her what she is--so absolutely straight and fearless. She sees love, and holds by what she believes its demands to be. I wouldn't wish her any different," he added loyally.

"Perhaps not. But if--supposing the man proves to have a wife already? He might be separated from her; Sara doesn't seem to know much about him. Or he may have a wife in a lunatic asylum who is likely to live for the next forty years. What then? Will Sara never marry if--if there were a circumstance like that--a really insurmountable obstacle?"

"No, I don't believe she will. I don't think she would wish to. If he loves her and she him, spiritually they would be bound to one another--lovers. And just the circumstance of his being tied to another woman would make no difference to Sara's point of view. She goes beyond material things--or the mere physical side of love."

"Then there is no chance for you unless Sara learns to *unlove* this man?"
Tim regarded her with faint amusement.

"Mother, do you think you could learn to unlove me--or my father?"
She laughed a little.

"You have me there, Tim," she acknowledged. "But"--hesitating a little--"Sara knows so little of the man, apparently, that she may have formed a mistaken estimate of his character. Perhaps he is not really the--the ideal individual she has pictured him."

Tim smiled.

"You are a very transparent person, mother mine," he said indulgently. "But I'm afraid your hopes of finding that the idol has feet of clay are predestined to disappointment."

"Have you met the man?" asked Elisabeth sharply.

"I do not even know his name. But I should imagine him a man of big, fine qualities."

"Since you don't know him, you can hardly pronounce an opinion."

A whimsical smile, touched with sadness, flitted across Tim's face.

"I know Sara," was all he said.

"Sara is given to idealizing the people she cares for," rejoined Elisabeth.

She spoke quietly, but her expression was curiously intent. It was as though she were gathering together her forces, concentrating them towards some definite purpose, veiled in the inscrutable depths of those strange eyes of hers.

"I find it difficult to forgive her," she said at last.

"That's not like you, mother."

"It is--just like me," she responded, a tone of half-tender mockery in her voice. "Naturally I find it difficult to forgive the woman who has hurt my son."

Tim answered her out of the fullness of the queer new wisdom with which love had endowed him.

"A man would rather be hurt by the woman he loves than humoured by the woman he doesn't love," he said quietly.

And Elisabeth, understanding, held her peace.

She had been very controlled, very wise and circumspect in her dealing with Tim, conscious of raw-edged nerves that would bear but the lightest of handling. But it was another woman altogether who, half-an-hour later, faced Geoffrey Durward in the seclusion of his study.

The two moving factors in Elisabeth's life had been, primarily, her love for her husband, and, later on, her love for Tim, and into this later love was woven all the passionately protective instinct of the maternal element. She was the type of woman who would have plucked the feathers from an archangel's wing if she thought they would contribute to her son's happiness; and now, realizing that the latter was threatened by the fact that his love for Sara had failed to elicit a responsive fire, she felt bitterly resentful and indignant.

"I tell you, Geoffrey," she declared in low, forceful tones, "she *shall* marry Tim--*she shall*! I will not have his beautiful young life marred and spoilt by the caprices of any woman."

Major Durward looked disturbed.

"My dear, I shouldn't call Sara in the least a capricious woman. She knows her own heart--"

"So does Tim!" broke in Elisabeth. "And, if I can compass it, he shall have his heart's desire."

Her husband shook his head.

"You cannot force the issue, my dear."

"Can I not? There's little a woman *cannot* do for husband or child! I tell you, Geoffrey--for you, or for Tim, to give you pleasure, to buy you happiness, I would sacrifice anybody in the world!"

She stood in front of him, her beautiful eyes glowing, and her voice was all shaken and a-thrill with the tumult of emotion that had gripped her. There was something about her which suggested a tigress on the defensive--at bay, shielding her young. Durward looked at her with kind, adoring eyes.

"That's beautiful of you, darling," he replied gently. "But it's a dangerous doctrine. And I know that, really, you're far too tender-hearted to sacrifice a fly."

Elisabeth regarded him oddly.

"You don't know me, Geoffrey," she said very slowly. "No man knows a woman, really--not all her thoughts." And had Major Durward, honest fellow, realized the volcanic force of passion hidden behind the tense inscrutability of his wife's lovely face, he would have been utterly confounded. We do not plumb the deepest depths even of those who are closest to us.

Civilisation had indeed forced the turgid river to run within the narrow channels hewn by established custom, but, released from the bondage of convention, the soul of Elisabeth Durward was that of sheer primitive woman, and the pivot of all her actions her love for her mate and for the man-child she had borne him.

Once, years ago, she had sacrificed justice, and honour, and a man's faith in womanhood on that same pitiless altar of love. But the story of that sacrifice was known only to herself and one other--and that other was not Durward.

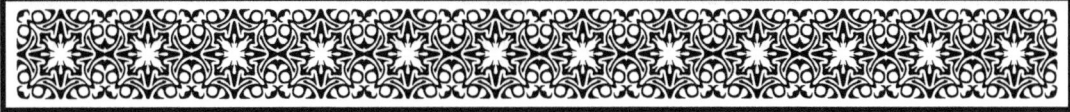

CHAPTER XXII
LOVE'S SACRAMENT

A full week had elapsed since the night of that eventful journey in pursuit of Molly, and from the moment when Garth had given Sara into the safe keeping of Jane Crab till the moment when he came upon her by the pergola at Rose Cottage, perched on the top of a ladder, engaged in tying back the exuberance of a Crimson Rambler, they had not met.

And now, as he halted at the foot of the ladder, Sara was conscious that her spirits had suddenly bounded up to impossible heights at the sight of the lean, dark face upturned to her.

"The Lavender Lady and Miles are pottering about in the greenhouse," she announced explanatorily, waving her hand in the direction of a distant glimmer of glass beyond the high box hedge which flanked the rose-garden.

"Are they?" Trent, thus arrested in the progress of his search for his host and hostess, seemed entirely indifferent as to whether it were ever completed or not. He leaned against one of the rose-wreathed pillars of the pergola and gazed negligently in the direction Sara indicated.

"How is Miss Molly?" he asked.

Sara twinkled.

"She is just beginning to discard sackcloth and ashes for something more becoming," she informed him gravely.

"That's good. Are you--are you all right after your tumble? I'm making these kind inquiries because, since it was my car out of which you elected to fall, I feel a sense of responsibility."

Sara descended from the ladder before she replied. Then she remarked composedly--

"It has taken precisely seven days, apparently, for that sense of responsibility to develop."

"On the contrary, for seven days my thirst for knowledge has been only restrained by the pointings of conscience."

"Then"--she spoke rather low--"was it conscience pointing you--away from Sunnyside?"

His hazel eyes flashed over her face.

"Perhaps it was--discretion," he suggested. "Looking in at shop windows when one has an empty purse is a poor occupation--and one to be avoided."

"Did you want to come?" she persisted gently.

Half absently he had cut off a piece of dead wood from the rose-bush next him and was twisting it idly to and fro between his fingers. At her words, the dead wood stem snapped suddenly in his clenched hand. For an instant he seemed about to make some passionate rejoinder. Then he slowly unclenched his hand and the broken twig fell to the ground.

"Haven't I made it clear to you--yet," he said slowly, "that what I want doesn't enter into the scheme of things at all?"

The brief speech held a sense of impending finality, and, in the silence which followed, the eyes of the man and woman met, questioned each other desperately, and answered.

There are moments when modesty is a false quantity, and when the big happinesses of life depend on a woman's capacity to realize this and her courage to act upon it. To Sara, it seemed that such a moment had come to her, and the absolute sincerity of her nature met it unafraid.

"No," she said quietly. "You have only made clear to me--what you want, Garth. Need we--pretend to each other any longer?"

"I don't understand," he muttered.

"Don't you?" She drew a littler nearer him, and the face she lifted to his was very white. But her eyes were shining. "That night--when I fell from the car--I--I wasn't unconscious."

For an instant he stared at her, incredulous. Then he swung aside a little, his hand gripping the pillar against which he had been leaning till his knuckles showed white beneath the straining skin.

"You--weren't unconscious?" he repeated blankly.

"No--not all the time. I--heard--what you said."

He seemed to pull himself together.

"Oh, Heaven only knows what I may have said at a moment like that," he answered carelessly, but his voice was rough and hoarse. "A man talks wild when the woman he's with only misses death by a hair's breath."

Sara's lips upturned at the corners in a slow smile--a smile that was neither mocking, nor tender, nor chiding, but an exquisite blending of all three. She caught her breath quickly--Trent could hear its soft sibilance. Then she spoke.

"Will you marry me, please, Garth?"

He drew back from her, violently, his underlip hard bitten. At last, after a long silence--

"No!" he burst out harshly. "No! I can't!"

For an instant she was shaken. Then, buoyed up by the memory of that night when she had lain in his arms and when the agony of the moment had stripped him of all power to hide his love, she challenged his denial.

"Why not?" Her voice was vibrant. "You love me!"

"Yes . . . I love you." The words seemed torn from him.

"Then why won't you marry me?"

It did not seem to her that she was doing anything unusual or unwomanly. The man she loved had carried his burden single-handed long enough. The time had come when for his own sake as well as for hers, she must wring the truth from him, make him break through the silence which had long been torturing them both. Whatever might be the outcome, whether pain or happiness, they must share it.

"Why won't you marry me, Garth?"

The little question, almost voiceless in its intensity, clamoured loudly at his heart.

"Don't tempt me!" he cried out hoarsely. "My God! I wonder if you know how you are tempting me?"

She came a little closer to him, laying her hand on his arm, while her great, sombre eyes silently entreated him.

As though the touch of her were more than he could bear, his hard-held passion crashed suddenly through the bars his will had set about it.

He caught her in his arms, lifting her sheer off her feet against his breast, whilst his lips crushed down upon her mouth and throat, burned against her white, closed lids, and the hard clasp of his arms about her was a physical pain--an exquisite agony that it was a fierce joy to suffer.

"Then--then you do love me?" She leaned against him, breathless, her voice unsteady, her whole slender body shaken with an answering passion.

"Love you?" The grip of his arms about her made response. "Love you? I love you with my soul and my body, here and through whatever comes Hereafter. You are my earth and heaven--the whole meaning of things--" He broke off abruptly, and she felt his arms slacken their hold and slowly unclasp as though impelled to it by some invisible force.

"What was I saying?" The heat of passion had gone out of his voice, leaving it suddenly flat and toneless. "'The whole meaning of things?'" He gave a curious little laugh. It had a strangled sound, almost like the cry of some tortured thing. "Then things *have* no meaning----"

Sara stood staring at him, bewildered and a little frightened.

"Garth, what is it?" she whispered. "What has happened?"

He turned, and, walking away from her a few paces, stood very still with his head bent and one hand covering his eyes.

Overhead, the sunshine, filtering in through the green trellis of leafy twigs, flaunted gay little dancing patches of gold on the path below, as the leaves moved flickeringly in the breeze, and where the twisted growth of a branch had left a leafless aperture, it flung a single shaft of quivering light athwart the pergola. It gleamed like a shining sword between the man and woman, as though dividing them one from the other and thrusting each into the shadows that lay on either hand.

"Garth----"

At the sound of her voice he dropped his hand to his side and came slowly back and stood beside her. His face was almost grey, and the tortured expression of his eyes seemed to hurt her like the stab of a knife.

"You must try to forgive me," he said, speaking very low and rapidly. "I had no earthly right to tell you that I cared, because--because I can't ask you to marry me. I told you once that I had forfeited my claim to the good things in life. That was true. And, having that knowledge, I ought to have kept away from you--for I knew how it was going to be with me from the first moment I saw you. I fought against it in the beginning--tried not to love you. Afterwards, I gave in, but I never dreamed that--you--would come to care, too. That seemed something quite beyond the bounds of human possibility."

"Did it? I can't see why it should?"

"Can't you?" He smiled a little. "If you were a man who has lived under a cloud for over twenty years, who has nothing in the world to recommend him, and only a tarnished reputation as his life-work, you, too, would have thought it inconceivable. Anyway, I did, and, thinking that, I dared to give myself the pleasure of seeing you--of being sometimes in your company. Perhaps"--grimly--"it was as much a torture as a joy on occasion. . . . But still, I was near you. . . . I could see you--touch your hand--serve you, perhaps, in any little way that offered. That was all something--something very wonderful to come into a life that, to all intents and purposes, was over. And I thought I could keep myself in hand--never let you know that I cared--"

"You certainly tried hard enough to convince me that you didn't," she interrupted ruefully.

"Yes, I tried. And I failed. And now, all that remains is for me to go away. I shall never forgive myself for having brought pain into your life--I, who would so gladly have brought only happiness. . . . God in Heaven!"--he whispered to himself as though the thought were almost blinding in the promise of ecstasy it held--"To have been the one to bring you happiness! . . ." He fell silent, his mouth wrung and twisted with pain.

Presently her voice came to him again, softly supplicating. "I shall never forgive you--if you go away and leave me," she added. "I can't do without you now--now that I know you care."

"But I **must** go! I can't marry you--you haven't understood--"

"Haven't I?" She smiled--a small, wise, wonderful smile that began somewhere deep in her heart and touched her lips and lingered in her eyes.

"Tell me," she said. "Are you married, Garth?"

He started.

"Married! God forbid!"

"And if you married me, would you be wronging any one?"

"Only you yourself," he answered grimly.

"Then nothing else matters. You are free--and I'm free. And I love you!"

She leaned towards him, her hands outheld, her mouth still touched with that little, mystic smile. "Please--tell me all over again now much you love me."

But no answering hands met hers. Instead, he drew away from her and faced her, stern-lipped.

"I must make you understand," he said. "You don't know what it is that you are asking. I've made shipwreck of my life, and I must pay the penalty. But, by God, I'm not going to let you pay it, too! And if you married me, you would have to pay. You would be joining your life to that of an outcast. I can never go out into the world as other men may. If I did"--slowly--"if I did, sooner or later I should be driven away--thrust back into my solitude. I have nothing to offer--nothing to give--only a life that has been cursed from the outset. Don't misunderstand me," he went on quickly. "I'm not complaining, bidding for your sympathy. If a man's a fool, he must be prepared to pay for his folly--even though it means a life penalty for a moment's madness. And I shall have to pay--to the uttermost farthing. Mine's the kind of debt which destiny never remits." He paused; then added defiantly: "The woman who married me would have to share in that payment--to go out with me into the desert in which I lie, and she would have to do this without knowing what she was paying for, or why the door of the world is locked against me. My lips are sealed, nor shall I ever be able to break the seal. *Now* do you understand why I can never ask you, or any other woman to be my wife?"

Sara looked at him curiously; he could not read the expression of her face.

"Have you finished?" she asked. "Is that all?"

"All? Isn't it enough?"--with a grim laugh.

"And you are letting this--this folly of your youth stand between us?"

"The world applies a harder word than folly to it!"

"I don't care anything at all about the world. What do *you* call it?"

He shrugged his shoulders.

"I call it folly to ask the criminal in the dock whether he approves the judge's verdict. He's hardly likely to!"

For a moment she was silent. Then she seemed to gather herself together.

"Garth, do you love me?"

The words fell clearly on the still, summer air.

"Yes"--doggedly--"I love you. What then?"

"What then? Why--this! I don't care what you've done. It doesn't matter to me whether you are an outcast or not. If you are, then I'm willing to be an outcast with you. Oh, Garth--My Garth! I've been begging you to marry me all afternoon, and--and----" with a broken little laugh--"you can't **keep on** refusing me!"

Before her passionate faith and trust the barriers he had raised between them came crashing down. His arms went round her, and for a few moments they clung together and love wiped out all bitter memories of the past and all the menace of the future.

But presently he came back to his senses. Very gently he put her from him.

"It's not right," he stammered unsteadily. "I can't accept this from you. Dear, you must let me go away. . . . I can't spoil your beautiful life by joining it to mine!"

She drew his arm about her shoulders again.

"You will spoil it if you go away. Oh! Garth, you dear, foolish man! When will you understand that love is the only thing that matters? If you had committed all the sins in the Decalogue, I shouldn't care! You're mine now"--jealously--"my lover. And I'm not going to be thrust out of your life for some stupid scruple. Let the past take care of itself. The present is ours. And--and I love you, Garth!"

It was difficult to reason coolly with her arms about him, her lips so near his own, and his great love for her pulling at his heart. But he made one further effort.

"If you should ever regret it, Sara?" he whispered. "I don't think I could bear that."

She looked at him with steady eyes.

"You will not have it to bear," she said. "I shall never regret it."

Still he hesitated. But the dawn of a great hope grew and deepened in his face.

"If you could be content to live here--at Far End . . . It is just possible!" He spoke reflectively, as though debating the matter with himself. "The curse has not followed me to this quiet little corner of the earth. Perhaps--after all . . . Sara, could you stand such a life? Or would you always be longing to get out into the great world? As I've told you, the world is shut to me. There's that in my past which blocks the way to any future. Have you the faith--the **courage**--to face that?"

Her eyes, steadfast and serene, met his.

"I have courage to face anything--with you, Garth. But I haven't courage to face living without you."

He bent his head and kissed her on the mouth--a slow, lingering kiss that held something far deeper and more enduring than mere passion. And Sara, as she kissed him back, her soul upon her lips, felt as though together they had partaken of love's holy sacrament.

"Beloved"--Garth's voice, unspeakably tender, came to her through the exquisite silence of the moment--"Beloved, it shall be as you wish. Whether I am right or wrong in taking this great gift you offer me--God knows! If I am wrong--then, please Heaven, whatever punishment there be may fall on me alone."

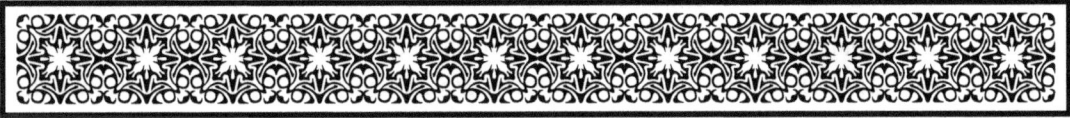

CHAPTER XXIII
A SUMMER IDYLL

The summer, of all seasons of the year, is very surely the perfect time for lovers, and to Sara the days that followed immediately upon her engagement to Garth Trent were days of unalloyed happiness.

These were wonderful hours which they passed together, strolling through the summer-foliaged woods, or lazing on the sun-baked sands, or, perhaps, roaming the range of undulating cliffs that stretched away to the west from the headland where Far End stood guard.

During those hours of intimate companionship, Sara began to learn the hidden deeps of Garth's nature, discovering the almost romantic delicacy of thought that underlay his harsh exterior.

"You're more than half a poet, my Garth!" she told him one day.

"A transcendental fool, in other words," he amended, smiling. "Well"--looking at her oddly--"perhaps you're right. But it's too late to improve me any. As the twig is bent, so the tree grows, you know."

"I don't want to improve you," Sara assured him promptly. "I shouldn't like you to be in the least bit different from what you are. It wouldn't be my Garth, then, at all."

So they would sit together and talk the foolish, charming nonsense that all lovers have talked since the days of Adam and Eve, whilst from above, the sun shone down and blessed them, and the waves, lapping peacefully on the shore, murmured an *obbligato* to their love-making.

Looking backward, in the bitter months that followed when her individual happiness had been caught away from her in a whirlwind of calamity, and when the whole world was reeling under the red storm of war, Sara could always remember the utter, satisfying peace of those golden days of early July--an innocent, un-thinking peace that neither she nor the world would ever quite regain. Afterwards, memory would always have her scarred and bitter place at the back of things.

Sara found no hardship now in receiving the congratulations of her friends--and they fell about her like rain--while in the long, intimate talks she had with Garth the fact that he would never speak of the past weighed with her not at all. She guessed that long ago he had been guilty of some mad, boyish escapade which, with his exaggerated sense of honour and the delicate idealism that she had learned to know as an intrinsic part of his temperamental make-up, he had magnified into a cardinal sin. And she was content to leave it at that and to accept the present, gathering up with both hands the happiness it held.

She had written to Elisabeth, telling her of her engagement, and, to her sur-prise, had received the most charming and friendly letter in return.

"Of course," wrote Elisabeth in her impulsive, flowing hand with its heavy dashes and fly-away dots, "we cannot but wish that it had been otherwise--that you could have learned to care for Tim--but you know better than any one of us where your happiness lies, and you are right to take it. And never think, Sara, that this is going to make any difference to our friendship. I could read between the lines of your letter that you had some such foolish thought in your mind. So little do I mean this to make any break between us that--as I can quite realize it would be too much to ask that you should come to us at Barrow just now--I propose coming down to Monkshaven. I want to meet the lucky individual who has won my Sara. I have not been too well lately--the heat has tried me--and Geoffrey is anxious that I should go away to the sea for a little. So that all things seem to point to my coming to Monkshaven. Does your primitive little village boast a hotel? Or, if not, can you engage some decent rooms for me?"

The remainder of the letter dealt with the practical details concerning the pro-posed visit, and Sara, in a little flurry of joyous excitement, had hurried off to the Cliff Hotel and booked the best suite of rooms it contained for Elisabeth.

On her way home she encountered Garth in the High Street, and forthwith proceeded to acquaint him with her news.

"I've just been fixing up rooms at the 'Cliff' for a friend of mine who is coming down here," she said, as he turned and fell into step beside her. "A woman friend," she added hastily, seeing his brows knit darkly.

"So much the better! But I could have done without the importation of any friends of yours--male or female--just now. They're entirely superfluous"--smiling.

"Well, I'm glad Mrs. Durward is coming, because--"

"*Who* did you say?" broke in Garth, pausing in his stride.

"Mrs. Durward--Tim's mother, you know," she explained. She had confided to him the history of her brief engagement to Tim.

Trent resumed his walk, but more slowly; the buoyancy seemed suddenly gone out of his step.

"Don't you think," he said, speaking in curiously measured tones, "that, in the circumstances, it will be a little awkward Mrs. Durward's coming here just now?"

Sara disclaimed the idea, pointing out that it was the very completeness of Elisabeth's conception of friendship which was bringing her to Monkshaven.

"When does she come?" asked Trent.

"On Thursday. I'm very anxious for you to meet her, Garth. She is so thoroughly charming. I think it is splendid of her not to let my broken engagement with Tim make any difference between us. Most mothers would have borne a grudge for that!"

"And you think Mrs. Durward has overlooked it?"--with a curious smile.

Sara enthusiastically assured him that this was the case.

"I wonder!" he said meditatively. "It would be very unlike Elis--unlike any woman"--he corrected himself hastily--"to give up a fixed idea so easily."

"Well"--Sara laughed gaily. "Nowadays you can't *compel* a person to marry the man she doesn't want--nor prevent her from marrying the man she does."

"I don't know. A determined woman can do a good deal."

"But Elisabeth isn't a bit the determined type of female you're evidently imagining," protested Sara, amused. "She is very beautiful and essentially feminine-- rather a wonderful kind of person, I think. Wait till you see her!"

"I'm afraid," said Trent slowly, "that I shall not see your charming friend. I have to run up to Town next week on--on business."

"Oh!" Sara's disappointment showed itself in her voice. "Can't you put it off?"

He halted outside a tobacconist's shop. "Do you mind waiting a moment while I go in here and get some baccy?"

He disappeared into the shop, and Sara stood gazing idly across the street, watching a jolly little fox-terrier enjoying a small but meaty bone he had filched from the floor of a neighbouring butcher's shop.

His placid enjoyment of the stolen feast was short-lived. A minute later a lean and truculent Irish terrier came swaggering round the corner, spotted the succulent morsel, and, making one leap, landed fairly on top of the smaller dog. In an instant pandemonium arose, and the quiet street re-echoed to the noise of canine combat.

The little fox-terrier put up a plucky fight in defence of his prior claim to the bone of contention, but soon superior weight began to tell, and it was evident that the Irishman was getting the better of the fray. The fox-terrier's owner, very elegantly dressed, watched the battle from a safe distance, wringing her hands and calling upon all and sundry of the small crowd which had speedily collected to save her darling from the lions.

No one, however, seemed disposed to relieve her of this office--for the Irishman was an ugly-looking customer--when suddenly, like a streak of light, a slim figure flashed across the road, and flung itself into the *melee*, whist a vibrating voice broke across the uproar with an imperative: "Let *go*, you brute!"

It was all over in a moment. Somehow Sara's small, strong hands had separated the twisting, growling, biting heap of dog into its component parts of fox and Irish, and she was standing with the little fox-terrier, panting and bleeding profusely, in her arms, while one or two of the bystanders--now that all danger was past--drove off the Irishman.

"Oh! But how *brave* of you!" The owner of the fox-terrier rustled forward. "I can't ever thank you sufficiently."

Sara turned to her, her black eyes blazing.

"Is this your dog?" she asked.

"Yes. And I'm sure"--volubly--"he would have been torn to pieces by that great hulking brute if you hadn't separated them. I should never have *dared*!"

Garth, coming out of the tobacconist's shop across the way, joined the little knot of people just in time to hear Sara answer cuttingly, as she put the terrier into its owner's arms--

"You've no business to *have* a dog if you've not got the pluck to look after him!"

As she and Trent bent their steps homeward, Sara regaled him with the full, true, and particular account of the dog-fight, winding up indignantly--

"Foul women like that ought not to be allowed to take out a dog licence. I hate people who shirk their responsibilities."

"You despise cowards?" he asked.

"More than anything on earth," she answered heartily.

He was silent a moment. Then he said reflectively--

"And yet, I suppose, a certain amount of allowance must be made for--nerves."

"It seems to me it depends on what your duty demands of you at the moment," she rejoined. "Nerves are a luxury. You can afford them when it makes no difference to other people whether you're afraid or not--but not when it does."

"And from what deeps did you draw such profound wisdom?" he asked quizzically.

Sara laughed a little.

"I had it well rubbed into me by my Uncle Patrick," she replied. "It was his *Credo*."

"And yet, I can understand any one's nerves cracking suddenly--after a prolonged strain."

"I don't think yours would," responded Sara contentedly, with a vivid recollection of their expedition to the island and its aftermath.

"Possibly not. But I suppose no man can be dead sure of himself--always."

"Will you come in?" asked Sara as they paused at Sunnyside gate.

"Not to-day, I think. I had better begin to accustom myself to doing without you, as I am going away so soon"--smiling.

"I wish you were not going," she rejoined discontentedly. "I so wanted you and Elisabeth to meet. *Must* you go?"

"I'm afraid I must. And it's better that I should go, on the whole. I should only be raging up and down like an untied devil because Mrs. Durward was taking up so much of your time! Let her have you to herself for a few days--and then, when I come back, I shall have you to *myself* again."

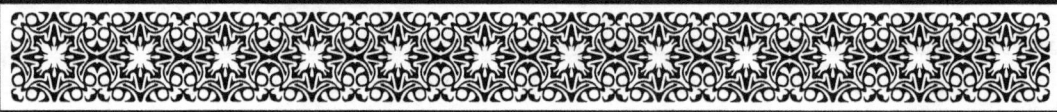

CHAPTER XXIV
PATCHES OF BLUE

Elisabeth frowned a little as she perused the letter which she had that morning received from Sara. It contained the information that rooms in her name had been booked at the Cliff Hotel, and further, that Sara was much disappointed that it would be impossible to arrange for her to meet Garth Trent, as he was leaving home on the Wednesday prior to her arrival.

Trent's departure was the last thing Elisabeth desired. Above all things, she wanted to meet the man whom she regarded as the stumbling-block in the path of her son, for if it were possible that anything might yet be done to further the desire of Tim's heart, it could only be if Elisabeth, as the *dea ex machina*, were acquainted with all the pieces in the game.

She must know what manner of man it was who had succeeded in winning Sara's heart before she could hope to combat his influence, and, if the feet of clay were there, she must see them herself before she could point them out to Sara's love-illusioned eyes. Should she fail of making Trent's acquaintance, she would be fighting in the dark.

Elisabeth pondered the matter for some time. Finally, she dispatched a telegram, prepaying a reply, to the proprietor of the Cliff Hotel, and a few hours later she announced to her husband that she proposed antedating her visit to Monkshaven by three days.

"I shall go down the day after to-morrow--on Monday," she said.

"Then I'd better send a wire to Sara," suggested Geoffrey.

"No, don't do that. I intend taking her by surprise." Elisabeth smiled and dimpled like a child in the possession of a secret. "I shall go down there just in time for dinner, and write to Sara the same evening."

Major Durward laughed with indulgent amusement.

"What an absurd lady you are still, Beth!" he exclaimed, his honest face beaming adoration. "No one would take you to be the mother of a grown-up son!"

"Wouldn't they?" For a moment Elisabeth's eyes--veiled, enigmatical as ever--rested on Tim's distant figure, where he stood deep in the discussion of some knotty point with the head gardener. Then they came back to her husband's face, and she laughed lightly. "Everybody doesn't see me through the rose-coloured spectacles that you do, dearest."

"There are no 'rose-coloured spectacles' about it," protested Geoffrey energetically. "No one on earth would take you for a day more than thirty--if it weren't for the solid fact of Tim's six feet of bone and muscle!"

Elisabeth jumped up and kissed her husband impulsively.

"Geoffrey, you're a great dear," she declared warmly. "Now I must run off and tell Fanchette to pack my things."

So it came about that on the following Tuesday, Sara, to her astonishment and delight, received a letter from Elisabeth announcing her arrival at the Cliff Hotel.

"Why, Elisabeth is already here!" she exclaimed, addressing the family at Sunnyside collectively. "She came last night."

Selwyn looked up from his correspondence with a kindly smile.

"That's good. You will be able, after all, to bring off the projected meeting between Mrs. Durward and your hermit--who, by the way, seems to have deserted his shell nowadays," he added, twinkling.

And Sara, blissfully unaware that in this instance Elisabeth had abrogated to herself the rights of destiny, responded smilingly--

"Yes. Fate has actually arranged things quite satisfactorily for once."

Half an hour later she presented herself at the Cliff Hotel, and was conducted upstairs to Mrs. Durward's sitting-room on the first floor.

Elisabeth welcomed her with all her wonted charm and sweetness. There was a shade of gravity in her manner as she spoke of Sara's engagement, but no hint of annoyance. She dwelt solely on Tim's disappointment and her own, exhibiting no bitterness, but only a rather wistful regret that another had succeeded where Tim had failed.

"And now," she said, drawing Sara out on to the balcony, where she had been sitting prior to the latter's arrival, "and now, tell me about the lucky man."

Sara found it a little difficult to describe the man she loved to the mother of the man she didn't love, but finally, by dint of skilful questioning, Elisabeth elicited the information she sought.

"Forty-three!" she exclaimed, as Sara vouchsafed his age. "But that's much too old for you, my dear!"

Sara shook her head.

"Not a bit," she smiled back.

"It seems so to me," persisted Elisabeth, regarding her with judicial eyes. "Somehow you convey such an impression of youth. You always remind me of spring. You are so slim and straight and vital--like a young sapling. However, perhaps Mr. Trent also has the faculty of youth. Youth isn't a matter of years, after all," she added contemplatively.

"Now go on," she commanded, after a moment. "Tell me what he looks like."

Sara laughed and plunged into a description of Garth's personal appearance.

"And he's got queer eyes--tawny-coloured like a dog's," she wound up, "with a quaint little patch of blue close to each of the pupils."

Elisabeth leaned forward, and beneath the soft laces of her gown the rise and fall of her breast quickened perceptibly.

"Patches of blue?" she repeated.

"Yes--it sounds as though the colours had run, doesn't it?" pursued Sara, laughing a little. "But it's really rather effective."

"And did you say his name was Trent--Garth Trent?" asked Elisabeth. She had gone a little grey about the mouth, and she moistened her lips with her tongue before speaking. There was a tone of incredulity in her voice.

"Yes. It's not a beautiful name, is it?" smiled Sara.

"It's rather a curious one," agreed Elisabeth with an effort. "I'm really quite longing to meet this odd man with the patchwork eyes and the funny name."

"You shall see him to-day," Sara promised. "Audrey Maynard is giving a picnic in Haven Woods, and Garth will be there. You will come with us, won't you?"

"I think I must," replied Elisabeth. "Although"--negligently--"picnics are not much in my line."

"Oh, Audrey's picnics aren't like other people's," rejoined Sara reassuringly.

"She runs them just as she runs everything else, on lines of combined perfection and informality! The lunch will be the production of a French chef, and the company a few carefully selected intimates."

"Very well, I'll come--if you're sure Mrs. Maynard won't object to the introduction of a complete stranger."

Sara regarded her affectionately.

"Have you ever met any one who 'objected' to you yet?" she asked with some amusement.

Elisabeth made no answer. Instead, she pointed to the Monk's Cliff, where the grey stone of Far End gleamed in the sunlight against its dark background of trees.

"Who lives there?" she asked. Sara's eyes followed the direction of her hand, and she smiled.

"*I'm* going to live there," she answered. "That's Garth's home."

"Oh-h!" Elisabeth drew a quick breath. "It's a grim-looking place," she added, after a moment. "Rather lonely, I should imagine."

"Garth is fond of solitude," replied Sara simply, and she missed the swift, searching glance instantly leveled at her by the hyacinth eyes.

When at length she took her departure, it was with a promise to return later on with Molly and Dr. Selwyn, so that they could all four walk out to Haven Woods together--since the doctor had undertaken to get through his morning's rounds in time to join the picnicking party.

Elisabeth accompanied her visitor to the head of the stairs, and then, returning to her room, stepped out on to the balcony once more. For a long time she stood leaning against the balustrade, gazing thoughtfully across the bay to that lonely house on the slope of the cliff.

"Garth Trent!" she murmured. "*Trent*! . . . And eyes with patches of blue in them! . . . Heavens! Can it possibly be? *Can* it be?"

There was a curious quality in her voice, a blending of incredulity and distaste, and yet something that savoured of satisfaction--almost of triumph.

Across her mental vision flitted a memory of just such eyes--gay, laughing, love-lit eyes, out of which the laughter had been suddenly dashed.

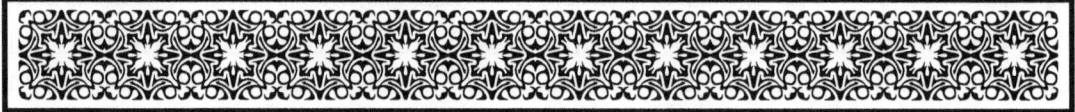

CHAPTER XXV
THE CUT DIRECT

It was a merry party which had gathered together in the shady heart of Haven Woods. The Selwyns, Sara and Elisabeth, Miles Herrick and the Lavender Lady were all there, and, in addition, there was a large and light-hearted contingent from Greenacres, where Audrey was entertaining a houseful of friends. Only Garth had not yet arrived.

Two young subalterns on leave and a couple of pretty American sisters, all of them staying at Greenacres, were making things hum, nobly seconded in their efforts by Miles Herrick, who had practically recovered from his sprained ankle and one of whose "good days" it chanced to be.

Every one seemed bubbling over with good-humour and high spirits, so that the dell re-echoed to the shouts of jolly laughter, while the birds, flitting nervously hither and thither, wondered what manner of creatures these were who had invaded their quiet sanctuary of the woods. And presently, when the whole party gathered round the white cloth, spread with every dainty that the inspired mind of Audrey's chef had been able to devise, and the popping corks began to punctuate the babble of chattering voices, they took wing and fled incontinently. They had heard similar sharp, explosive sounds before, and had noted them as being generally the harbingers of sudden death.

"Where's that wretched hermit of yours, Sara?" demanded Audrey gaily. "I told him we should lunch at one, and it's already a quarter-past. Ah!"--catching sight of a lean, supple figure advancing between the trees--"Here he is at last!"

A shout greeted Garth's approach, and the uproarious quartette composed of the two subalterns and the girls from New York City pounded joyously with their forks upon their plates, creating a perfect pandemonium of noise, Miles recklessly participating in the clamorous welcome, while the Lavender Lady fluttered her handkerchief, and Sara and Audrey both hurried forward to meet the late comer. In the general excitement nobody chanced to observe the effect which Trent's appearance had had upon one of the party.

Elisabeth had half-risen from the grassy bank on which she had been sitting, and her face was suddenly milk-white. Even her lips had lost their soft rose-colour, and were parted as if an exclamation of some kind had been only checked from passing them by sheer force of will.

Out of her white face, her eyes, seeming so dark that they were almost violet, stared fixedly at Garth as he approached. Their expression was as masked, as enigmatical as ever, yet back of it there gleamed an odd light, and it was as though some curious menace lay hidden in its quiet, slumbrous fire.

The little group composed of Audrey, Sara, and Garth had joined the main party now, and Garth was shaking eager, outstretched hands and laughingly tossing back the shower of chaff which greeted his tardy arrival.

Then Sara, laying her hand on his arm, steered him towards Elisabeth. Some one who had been standing a little in front of the latter, screening her from Trent's view, moved aside as they approached.

"Garth, let me introduce you to Mrs. Durward."

The smile that would naturally have accompanied the words was arrested ere it dawned, and involuntarily Sara drew back before the instant, startling change in Garth's face. It had grown suddenly ashen, and his eyes were like those of a man who, walking in some pleasant place, finds all at once, that a bottomless abyss has opened at his feet.

For a full moment he and Elisabeth stared at each other in a silence so vital, so pregnant with some terrible significance, that it impacted upon the whole prevailing atmosphere of care-free jollity.

A sudden muteness descended on the party, the laughing voices trailing off into affrighted silence, and in the dumb stillness that followed Sara was vibrantly conscious of the hostile clash of wills between the man and woman who had, in a single instant, become the central figures of the little group.

Then Elisabeth's voice--that amazingly sweet voice of hers--broke the profound quiet.

"Mr.--Trent"--she hesitated delicately before the name--"and I have met before."

And quite deliberately, with a proud, inflexible dignity, she turned her back upon him and moved away.

Sara never forgot the few moments that followed. She felt as though she were on the brink of some crisis in her life which had been slowly drawing nearer and nearer to her and was now acutely imminent, and instinctively she sought to gather all her energies together to meet it. What it might be she could not guess, but she was sure that this declared enmity between the man she loved and the woman who was her friend preluded some menace to her happiness.

Her eyes sought Garth's in horror-stricken interrogation.

"What is it? What does she mean?" she demanded swiftly, in a breathless undertone, instinctively drawing aside from the rest of the party.

He laughed shortly.

"She means mischief, probably," he replied. "Mrs. Durward is no friend of mine."

Sara's eyes blazed.

"She shall explain," she exclaimed impetuously, and she swung aside, meaning to follow Elisabeth and demand an explanation of the insult. But Garth checked her.

"No," he said decidedly. "Please do nothing--say nothing. For Audrey's sake we can't have a scene--here."

"But it's unpardonable----"

"Do as I say," he insisted. "Believe me, you will only make things worse if you interfere. I will make my apologies to Audrey and go. For my sake, Sara"--he looked at her intently--"go back and face it out. Behave as if nothing had happened."

Compelled, in spite of herself, by his insistence, Sara reluctantly assented and, leaving him, made her way slowly back to the others.

A disjointed buzz of talk sprayed up against her ears. Every one rushed into conversation, making valiant, if quite fruitless efforts to behave as though nothing out of the ordinary had occurred, while, a little apart from the main group, Elisabeth stood alone.

Meanwhile Trent sought out his hostess, and together they moved away, pausing at last beneath the canopy of trees.

"No words can quite meet what has just occurred," he said formally. "I can only express my regret that my presence here should have occasioned such a *contretemps*."

Although the whole brief scene had been utterly incomprehensible to her, Audrey intuitively sensed the bitter hurt underlying the harshly spoken words, and the outraged hostess was instantly submerged in the friend.

"I am so sorry about it, Garth," she said gently, "although, of course, I don't understand Mrs. Durward's behaviour."

"That is very kind of you!" he replied, his voice softening. "But please do not visit your very natural indignation upon Mrs. Durward. I alone am to blame, I ought never to have renounced my role of hermit. Unfortunately"--with a brief smile of such sadness that Audrey felt her heart go out to him in a sudden rush of sympathy--"my mere presence is an abuse of my friends' hospitality."

"No, no!" she exclaimed quickly. "We are all glad to have you with us--we were so pleased when--when at last you came out of your shell, Garth"--with a faint smile.

"Still the fact remains that I am outside the social pale. I had no business to thrust myself in amongst you. However--after this--you may rest assured that I shan't offend again."

"I decline to rest assured of anything of the kind," asserted Audrey with determination. "Don't be such a fool, Garth--or so unfair to your friends. Just because you chance to have met a women who, for some reason, chooses to cut you, doesn't alter our friendship for you in the very least. What Mrs. Durward may have against you I don't know--and I don't care either. *I* have nothing against you, and I don't propose to give any pal of mine the go-by because some one else happens to have quarreled with him."

Trent's eyes were curiously soft as he answered her.

"Thank you for that," he said earnestly. "All the same, I think you will have to make up your mind to allow your--friend, as you are good enough to call me, to go to the wall. You, and others like you, dragged him out, but, believe me, his place is not in the centre of the room. There are others besides Mrs. Durward who would give you the reason why, if you care to know it."

"I don't care to know it," responded Audrey firmly. "In fact, I should decline to recognize any reason against my calling you friend. I don't intend to let you go, nor will Miles, you'll find."

"Ah! Herrick! He's a good chap, isn't he?" said Trent a little wistfully.

"We all are--once you get to know us," returned Audrey, persistently cheerful. "And Sara--Sara won't let you go either, Garth."

His sensitive, bitter mouth twisted suddenly.

"If you don't mind," he said quickly, "we won't talk about Sara. And I won't keep you any longer from your guests. It was--just like you--to take it as you have done, Audrey. And if, later on, you find yourself obliged to revise your opinion of me--I shall understand. And I shall not resent it."

"I'm not very likely to do what you suggest."

He looked at her with a curious expression on his face.

"I'm afraid it is only too probable," he rejoined simply.

He wrung her hand, and, turning, walked swiftly away through the wood, while Audrey retraced her footsteps in the direction of the dell.

She was feeling extremely annoyed at what she considered to be Mrs. Durward's hasty and inconsiderate action. It was unpardonable of any one thus to spoil the harmony of the day, she reflected indignantly, and then she looked up and met Elisabeth's misty, hyacinth eyes, full of a gentle, appealing regret.

"Mrs. Maynard, I must beg you to try and pardon me," she said, approaching with a charming gesture of apology. "I have no excuse to offer except that Mr. Trent is a man I--I cannot possibly meet." She paused and seemed to swallow with some difficulty, and of a sudden Audrey was conscious of a thrill of totally unexpected compassion. There was so evidently genuine pain and emotion behind the hesitating apology.

"I am sorry you should have been distressed," she replied kindly. "It has been a most unfortunate affair all round."

Elisabeth bestowed a grateful little smile upon her.

"If you will forgive me," she said, "I will say good-bye now. I am sure you will understand my withdrawing."

"Oh no, you mustn't think of such a thing," cried Audrey hospitably, though within herself she could not but acknowledge that the suggestion was a timely one.

"Please don't run away from us like that."

"It is very kind of you, but really--if you will excuse me--I think I would prefer not to remain. I feel somewhat ***bouleversee***. And I am so distressed to have been the unwitting cause of spoiling your charming party."

Audrey hesitated.

"Of course, if you would really rather go----" she began.

"I would rather," persisted Elisabeth with a gentle inflexibility of purpose. "Will you give a message to Sara for me?" Audrey nodded. "Ask her to come and see me to-morrow, and tell her that--that I will explain." Suddenly she stretched out an impulsive hand. "Oh, Mrs. Maynard! If you knew how much I dread explaining this matter to Sara! Perhaps, however"--her eyes took on a thoughtful expression--"Perhaps, however, it may not be necessary--perhaps it can be avoided."

A sense of foreboding seemed to close round Audrey's heart, as she met the gaze of the beautiful, enigmatic eyes. What was it that Elisabeth intended to "explain" to Sara? Something connected with Garth Trent, of course, and it was impossible, in view of the attitude Elisabeth had assumed, to hope that it could be aught else than something to his detriment.

"If an explanation can be avoided, Mrs. Durward," she said rather coldly, "I think it would be much better. The least said, the soonest mended, you know," she added, looking straight into the baffling eyes.

The two women, all at once antagonistic and suspicious of each other, shook hands formally, and Elisabeth took her way through the woods, while Audrey rejoined her neglected guests and used her best endeavours to convert an entertainment that threatened to become a failure into, at least, a qualified success. By dint of infinite tact, and the loyal cooperation of Miles Herrick, she somehow achieved it, and the majority of the picnickers enjoyed themselves immensely.

Only Sara felt as though a shadow had crept out from some hidden place and cast its grey length across the path whereon she walked, while Miles and Audrey, discerning the shadow with the clear-sighted vision of friendship, were filled with apprehension for the woman whom they had both learned to love.

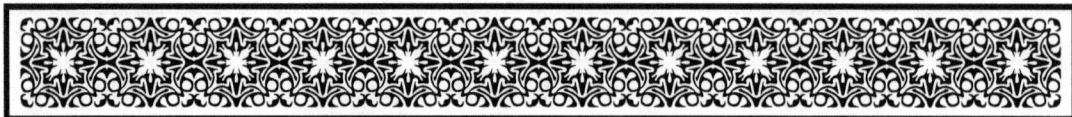

CHAPTER XXVI
A MIDNIGHT VISITOR

Judson crossed the hall at Far End and, opening the front door, peered anxiously out into the moonlit night for the third time that evening.

Neither he nor his wife could surmise what had become of their master. He had gone away, as they knew, with the intention of joining a picnic party in Raven Woods, but he had given no instructions that he wished the dinner-hour postponed, and now the beautiful little dinner which Mrs. Judson had prepared and cooked for her somewhat exigent employer had been entirely robbed of its pristine delicacy of flavour, since it had been "keeping hot" in the oven for at least two hours.

"Coming yet?" queried Mrs. Judson, as her husband returned to the kitchen.

The latter shook his head.

"Not a sign of 'im," he replied briefly.

Ten minutes later, the house door opened and closed with a bang, and Judson hastened upstairs to ascertain his master's wishes. When he again rejoined the wife of his bosom, his face wore a look of genuine concern.

"Something's happened," he announced solemnly. "Ten years have I been in Mr. Trent's service, and never, Maria, never have I seen him look as he do now."

"What's he looking like, then?" demanded Mrs. Judson, pausing with a saucepan in her hand.

"Like a man what's been in hell," replied her husband dramatically. "He's as white as that piece of paper"--pointing to the sheet of cooking paper with which Mrs. Judson had been conscientiously removing the grease from the chipped potatoes. "And his eyes look wild. He's been walking, too--must have walked twenty miles or thereabouts, I should think, for he seems dead beat and his boots are just a mask of mud. His coat's torn and splashed, as well--as if he'd pushed his way through bushes and all, without ever stopping to see where he was going."

"Then he'll be wanting his dinner," observed Mrs. Judson practically. "I'll dish it up--'tisn't what you might call actually spoiled as yet."

"He won't have any. 'Judson,' he says to me, 'bring me a whisky-and-soda and some sandwiches. I don't want nothing else. And then you can lock up and go to bed.'"

"Well, then, bless the man, look alive and get the whisky-and-soda and a tray ready whiles I cut the sandwiches," exclaimed the excellent Mrs. Judson promptly, giving her bemused spouse a push in the direction of the pantry and herself bustling away to fetch a loaf of bread.

"Right you are. But I was so took aback at the master's appearance, Maria, you could have knocked me down with a feather. I wonder if his young lady's given him his congy?" he added reflectively.

Mrs. Judson did not stay to discuss the question, but set about preparing the sandwiches, and a few minutes later Judson carried into Trent's own particular snuggery an attractive-looking little tray and placed it on a table at his master's elbow.

The man had not been far out in his reckoning when he opined that his master had walked "twenty miles or thereabouts." When he had quitted Haven Woods, Garth had started off, heedless of the direction he took, and, since then, he had been tramping, almost blindly, up hill and down dale, over hedges, through woods, along the shore, stumbling across the rocks, anywhere, anywhere in the world to get away from the maddening, devil-ridden thoughts which had pursued him since the brief meeting with a woman whose hyacinth eyes recalled the immeasurable anguish of years ago and threatened the joy which the future seemed to promise.

His face was haggard. Heavy lines had graved themselves about his mouth, and beneath drawn brows his eyes glowed like sombre fires.

Judson paused irresolutely beside him.

"Shall I pour you out a whisky, sir?" he inquired.

Trent started. He had been oblivious of the man's entrance.

"No. I'll do it myself--presently. Lock up and go to bed," he answered brusque-ly.

But Judson still hesitated. There was an expression of affectionate solicitude on his usually wooden face.

"Better have one at once, sir," he said persuasively. "And I think you'll find the chicken sandwiches very good, sir, if you'll excuse my mentioning it."

For a moment a faint, kindly smile chased away the look of intense weariness in Garth's eyes.

"You transparent old fool, Judson!" he said indulgently. "You're like an old hen clucking round. Very well, make me a whisky, if you will, and give me one of those superlative sandwiches."

Judson waited on him contentedly.

"Anything more to-night, sir? Shall I close the window?" with a gesture towards the wide-open window near which his master sat.

Garth shook his head, and, when at last the manservant had reluctantly taken his departure, he remained for a long time sitting very still, staring out across the moon-washed garden.

Presently he stirred restlessly. Glancing round the room, his eyes fell on his violin, lying upon the table with the bow beside it just as he had laid it down that morning after he had been improvising, in a fit of mad spirits, some variations on the theme of Mendelssohn's Wedding March.

He took up the instrument and struck a few desultory chords. Then, tucking it more closely beneath his chin, he began to play--a broken, fitful melody of haunting sadness, tormented by despairing chords, swept hither and thither by rushing minor cadences--the very spirit of pain itself, wandering, ghost-like, in desert places.

Upstairs Judson turned heavily in his bed.

"Just hark to 'im, Maria," he muttered uneasily. "He fair makes my flesh creep with that doggoned fiddle of his. 'Tis like a child crying in the dark. I wish he'd stop."

But the sad strains still went on, rising and falling, while Garth paced back and forth the length of the room and the candles flickered palely in the moonlight that poured in through the open window.

Suddenly, across the lawn a figure flitted, noiseless as a shadow. It paused once, as though listening, then glided forward again, slowly drawing nearer and nearer until at last it halted on the threshold of the room.

Garth, for the moment standing with his back towards the window, continued playing, oblivious of the quiet listener. Then, all at once, the feeling that he was no longer alone, that some one was sharing with him the solitude of the night, invaded his consciousness. He turned swiftly, and as his glance fell upon the silent figure standing at the open window, he slowly drew his violin from beneath his chin and remained staring at the apparition as though transfixed.

It was a woman who had thus intruded on his privacy. A scarf of black lace was twisted, hood-like, about her head, and beneath its fragile drapery was revealed the beautiful face and haunting, mysterious eyes of Elisabeth Durward. She had flung a long black cloak over her evening gown, and where it had fallen a little open at the throat her neck gleamed privet-white against its shadowy darkness.

The mystical, transfiguring touch of the moon's soft light had eliminated all signs of maturity, investing her with an amazing look of youth, so that for an instant it seemed to Trent as though the years had rolled back and Elisabeth Eden, in all the incomparable beauty of her girlhood, stood before him.

He gazed at her in utter silence, and the brooding eyes returned his gaze un-flinchingly.

"Good God!"

The words burst from him at last in a low, tense whisper, and, as if the sound broke some spell that had been holding both the man and woman motionless, Elisa-beth stepped across the threshold and came towards him.

Trent made a swift gesture--almost, it seemed, a gesture of aversion.

"Why have you come here?" he demanded hoarsely.

She drew a little nearer, then paused, her hand resting on the table, and looked at him with a strange, questioning expression in her eyes.

"This is a poor welcome, Maurice," she observed at last.

He winced sharply at the sound of the name by which she had addressed him, then, recovering himself, faced her with apparent composure.

"I have no welcome for you," he said in measured tones. "Why should I have? All that was between us two . . . ended . . . half a life-time ago."

"No!" she cried out. "No! Not all! There is still my son's happiness to be reck-oned."

"Your son's happiness?" He stared at her amazedly. "What has your son's happiness to do with me?"

"Everything!" she answered. "Everything! Sara Tennant is the woman he loves."

"And have you come here to blame me for the fact that she does not return his love?"--with an accent of ironical amusement.

"No, I don't blame you. But if it had not been for you she would have married him. They were engaged, and then"--her voice shook a little--"you came! You came--and robbed Tim of his happiness."

Trent smiled sarcastically.

"An instance of the grinding of the mills of God," he said lightly. "You robbed me--you'll agree?--of something I valued. And now--inadvertently--I have robbed you in return of your son's happiness. It appears"--consideringly--"an unusually just dispensation of Providence. And the sins of the parents are visited on the child, as is the usual inscrutable custom of such dispensations."

Elisabeth seemed to disregard the bitter gibe his speech contained. She looked at him with steady eyes.

"I want you--out of the way," she said deliberately.

"Indeed?" The indifferent, drawling tone was contradicted by the sudden dangerous light that gleamed in the hazel eyes. "You mean you want me--to pay--once more?"

She looked away uneasily, flushing a little.

"I'm afraid it does amount to that," she admitted.

"And how would you suggest it should be done?" he inquired composedly.

Her eyes came back to his face. There was an eager light in them, and when she spoke the words hurried from her lips in imperative demand.

"Oh, it would be so easy, Maurice! You have only to convince Sara that you are not fit to marry her--or any woman, for that matter! Tell her what your reputation is--tell her why you can never show yourself amongst your fellow men, why you live here under an assumed name. She won't want to marry you when she knows these things, and Tim would have his chance to win her back again."

"You mean--let me quite understand you, Elisabeth"--Trent spoke with curious precision--"that I am to blacken myself in Sara's eyes, so that, discovering what a wolf in sheep's clothing I am, she will break off our engagement. That, I take it, is your suggestion?"

Beneath his searching glance she faltered a moment. Then--

"Yes," she answered boldly. "That is it."

"It's a charming programme," he commented. "But it doesn't seem to me that you have considered Sara at all in the matter. It will hardly add to her happiness to find that she has given her heart to--what shall we say?"--smiling disagreeably--"to the wrong kind of man?"

"Of, of course, she will be upset, *disillusionnee*, for a time. She will suffer. But then we all have our share of suffering. Sara cannot hope to be exempt. And afterwards--afterwards"--her eyes shining--"she will be happy. She and Tim will be happy together."

"And so you are prepared to cause all this suffering, Sara's and mine--though I suppose"--with a bitter inflection--"that last hardly counts with you!--in order to secure Tim's happiness?"

"Yes," significantly, "I am prepared--to do anything to secure that."

Trent stared at her in blank amazement.

"Have you *no* conscience?" he asked at last. "Have you never had any?"

She looked at him a little piteously.

"You don't understand," she muttered. "You don't understand. I'm his mother. And I want him to be happy."

He shrugged his shoulders.

"I am sorry," he said, "that I cannot help you. But I'm afraid Tim's happiness isn't going to be purchased at my expense. I haven't the least intention of blackening myself in the eyes of the woman I love for the sake of Tim--or of twenty Tims. Please understand that, once and for all."

He gestured as though to indicated that she should precede him to the window by which she had entered. But she made no movement to go. Instead she flung back her cloak as though it were stifling her, and caught him impetuously by the arm.

"Maurice! Maurice! For God's sake, listen to me!" Her voice was suddenly shaken with passionate entreaty. "Use some other method, then! Break with her some other way! If you only knew how I hate to ask you this--I who have already brought only sorrow and trouble into your life! But Tim--my son--he must come first!" She pressed a little closer to him, lifting her face imploringly. "Maurice, you loved me once--for the sake of that love, grant me my boy's happiness!"

Quietly, inexorably, he disengaged himself from the eager clasp of her hand. Her beautiful, agonized face, the vehement supplication of her voice, moved him not a jot.

"You are making a poor argument," he said coldly. "You are making your request in the name of a love that died three-and-twenty years ago."

"Do you mean"--she stared at him--"that you have not cared--at all--since?" She spoke incredulously. Then, suddenly, she laughed. "And I--what a fool I was!--I used to grieve--often--thinking how you must be suffering!"

He smiled wryly as at some bitter memory.

"Perhaps I did," he responded shortly. "Death has its pains--even the death of first love. My love for you died hard, Elisabeth--but it died. You killed it."

"And you will not do what I ask for the sake of the love you--once--gave me?" There was a desperate appeal in her low voice.

He shook his head. "No," he said, "I will not."

She made a gesture of despair.

"Then you drive me into doing what I hate to do!" she exclaimed fiercely. She was silent for a moment, standing with bowed head, her mouth working painfully. Then, drawing herself up, she faced him again. There was something in the lithe, swift movement that recalled a panther gathering itself together for its spring.

"Listen!" she said. "If you will not find some means of breaking off your engagement with Sara, then I shall tell her the whole story--tell her what manner of man it is she proposes to make her husband!"

There was a supreme challenge in her tones, and she waited for his answer defiantly--her head flung back, her whole body braced, as it were, to resistance.

In the silence that followed, Trent drew away from her--slowly, repugnantly, as though from something monstrous and unclean.

"You wouldn't--you *couldn't* do such a thing!" he exclaimed in low, appalled tones of unbelief.

"I could!" she asserted, though her face whitened and her eyes flinched beneath his contemptuous gaze.

"But it would be a vile thing to do," he pursued, still with that accent of incredulous abhorrence. "Doubly vile for *you* to do this thing."

"Do you think I don't know that--don't realize it?" she answered desperately. "You can say nothing that could make me think it worse than I do already. It would be the basest action of which any woman could be guilty. I recognize that. And yet"--she thrust her face, pinched and strained-looking, into his--"***and yet I shall do it***. I'd take that sin--or any other--on my conscience for the sake of Tim."

Trent turned away from her with a gesture of defeat, and for a moment or two he paced silently backwards and forwards, while she watched him with burning eyes.

"Do you realize what it means?" she went on urgently. "You have no way out. You can't deny the truth of what I have to tell."

"No," he acknowledged harshly. "As you say, I cannot deny it. No one knows that better than yourself."

Suddenly he turned to her, and his face was that of a man in uttermost anguish of soul. Beads of moisture rimmed his drawn mouth, and when he spoke his voice was husky and uneven.

"Haven't I suffered enough--paid enough?" he burst out passionately. "You've had your pound of flesh. For God's sake, be satisfied with that! Leave--Garth Trent--to build up what is left of his life in peace!"

The roughened, tortured tones seemed to unnerve her. For a moment she hid her face in her hands, shuddering, and when she raised it again the tears were running down her cheeks.

"I can't--I can't!" she whispered brokenly. "I wish I could . . . you were good to me once. Oh! Maurice, I'm not a bad woman, not a wicked woman . . . but I've my son to think of . . . his happiness." She paused, mastering, with an effort, the emotion that threatened to engulf her. "Nothing else counts--***nothing***! If you go to the wall, Tim wins."

"So I'm to pay--first for your happiness, and now, more than twenty years later, for your son's. You don't ask--very much--of a man, Elisabeth."

He had himself in hand now. The momentary weakness which had wrenched that brief, anguished appeal from his lips was past, and the dry scorn of his voice cut like a lash, stinging her into hostility once more.

"I have given you the chance to break with Sara yourself--on any pretext you choose to invent," she said hardly. "You've refused--" She hesitated. "You do--still refuse, Maurice?" Again the note of pleading, of appeal in her voice. It was as though she begged of him to spare them both the consequences of that refusal.

He bowed. "Absolutely."

She sighed impatiently.

"Then I must take the only other way that remains. You know what that will be."

He stooped, and, picking up her cloak which had fallen to the floor, held it for her to put on. He had completely regained his customary indifference of manner.

"I think we need not prolong this interview, then," he said composedly.

Elisabeth drew the cloak around her and moved slowly towards the window. Outside, the tranquil moonlight still flooded the garden, the peaceful quiet of the night remained all undisturbed by the fierce conflict of human wills and passions that had spent itself so uselessly.

"One thing more"--she paused on the threshold as Trent spoke again--"You will not blacken the name of--"

"*No*!" It was as though she had struck the unuttered word from his lips. "Did you think I should? Those who bear it have suffered enough. There's no need to drag it through the mire a second time."

With a quick movement she drew her cloak more closely about her, and stepped out into the garden. For a moment Garth watched her crossing the lawns, a slender, upright, swiftly moving shadow. Then a clump of bushes, thrusting its wall of darkness into the silver sea of moonlight, hid her from his sight, and he turned back into the room. Stumblingly he made his way to the chimney-piece, and, resting his arms upon it, hid his face.

For a long time he remained thus, motionless, while the grandfather clock in the corner ticked away indifferently, and one by one the candles guttered down and went out in little pools of grease.

When at last he raised his face, it looked almost ghastly in the moonlight, so lined and haggard was it, and its sternly set expression was that of a man who had schooled himself to endure the supreme ill that destiny may hold in store.

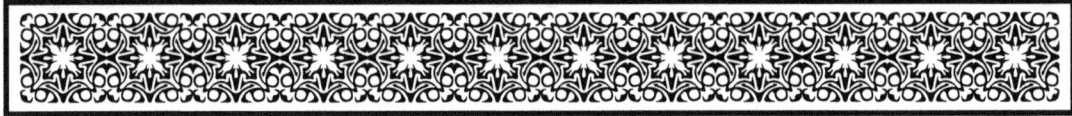

CHAPTER XXVII
J'ACCUSE!

O f course, there could be but one ending to it all. The man to whom you have promised yourself--Garth Trent--was court-martialled and cashiered."

As she finished speaking, Elisabeth's hands, which had been tightly locked together upon her knee, relaxed and fell stiffly apart, cramped with the intensity of their convulsive pressure.

Sara sat silent, staring with unseeing eyes across the familiar bay to that house on the cliff where lived the man whose past history--that history he had guarded so strenuously and completely from the ears of their little world--had just been revealed to her.

Mentally she was envisioning the whole scene of the story which hesitatingly--almost unwilling, it seemed--Elisabeth had poured out. She could see the lonely fort on the Indian Frontier, sparsely held by its indomitable little band of British soldiers, and ringed about on every side by the hill tribes who had so suddenly and unexpectedly risen in open rebellion. In imagination she could sense the hideous tension as day succeeded day and each dawning brought no sign of the longed-for relief forces. Indeed, it was not even known if the messengers sent by the officer in command had got safely through to the distant garrison to deliver his urgent message asking succour. And each evening found those who were besieged within the fort with diminished rations, and diminished hope, and with one or more dead to mark the enemy's unceasing vigilance.

And then had come the mysterious apparent withdrawal of the tribesmen. For hours no sign of the enemy had been seen, nor a single fugitive shot fired when one or other of the besieged had risked themselves at an unguarded aperture, whereas, until that morning, for a man to show himself, even for a moment, had been to court almost certain death.

Could the rebels have received word of the approach of a relieving force, whispers of a punitive expedition on its way, and so stolen stealthily, discreetly away in the silence of the night?

The hearts of the little beleaguered force rose high with hope, but again morning drew to evening without bringing sight or sound of succour. Only the enemy persisted in that strange, unbroken silence, and, at last, a hasty council of war was held within the fort, and Garth Trent, together with a handful of men, had been detailed to make a reconnaissance.

Sara could picture the little party stealing out on their dangerous errand--dangerous, indeed, if the withdrawal of the tribesmen were but a bluff, a scheme devised to lull the besieged into a false sense of security in order to attack them later at a greater disadvantage. And then--the sudden spit of a rifle, a ringing fusillade of shots in the dense darkness! The reconnaissance party had run into an ambuscade!

Sara could guess well the frayed nerves, the low vitality of men who were short of food, short of sleep, and worn with incessant watching night and day. But--Could it be possible that Englishmen had flinched at the crucial moment--lost their nerve and fled in wild disorder? Englishmen--who held the sacred trust of empire in their hands--to show the white feather to a horde of rebel natives! It was inconceivable! Sara, reared in the great tradition by that gallant gentleman, Patrick Lovell, refused to credit it.

She drew a long, shuddering breath.

"I don't believe it," she said.

Elisabeth looked at her with a pitying comprehension of the blow she had just dealt her.

"I'm afraid," she said gently, almost deprecatingly, "that there is no questioning the finding of the court-martial. Garth must have lost his head at the unexpectedness of the attack. And panic is a curious, unaccountable kind of thing, you know."

"I don't believe it," reiterated Sara stubbornly.

Elisabeth bent forward.

"My dear," she said, "there is no possibility of doubt. Garth was wounded; they brought him in afterwards--***shot in the back***! . . . Oh! It was all a horrible business! And the most wretched part of it all was that in reality they were only a few stray tribesmen whom our men had encountered. Perhaps Garth thought they were outnumbered--I don't know. But anyway, coming on the top of all that had gone before, the surprise attack in the darkness broke his nerve completely. He didn't even attempt to make a stand. He simply gave way. What followed was just a headlong scramble as to who could save his skin first! I shall never forget Garth's return after--after the court-martial." She shuddered a little at the memory. "I--I was engaged to him at the time, Sara, and I had no choice but to break it off. Garth was cashiered--disgraced--done for."

Sara's drooping figure suddenly straightened.

"*You--you*--were engaged to Garth?" she said in a queer, high voice.

"Yes"--simply. "I had promised to marry him."

Sara was silent for a long moment. Then--

"He never told me," she muttered. "He never told me."

"No? It was hardly likely he would, was it? He couldn't tell you that without telling you--the rest."

Sara made no answer. She felt stunned--beaten into helpless silence by the quiet, inexorable voice that, bit by bit, minute by minute, had drawn aside the veil of ignorance and revealed the dry bones and rottenness that lay hidden behind it.

"I don't believe it!" she had cried in a futile effort to convince herself by the sheer reiteration of denial. But she *did* believe it, nevertheless. The whole miserable story tallied too accurately with the bitterly significant remarks that Garth himself had let fall from time to time.

That day of the dog-fight, for instance. What was it he had said? "*A certain amount of allowance must be made for nerves*."

And again: "*I suppose no man can be dead sure of himself--always*."

The implication was too horribly clear to be evaded.

He had told her, moreover, that he was a man who had made a shipwreck of his life, that in a moment of folly--a moment of funk she knew now to be the veridical description!--he had flung away the whole chances of his life. The man whom she had loved, and, in her love, idealized, had proved himself, when the test came, that most despicable of things, a coward! The pain of realization was almost unbearable.

Suddenly, across the utter desolation of the moment there shot a single ray of hope. She turned triumphantly to Elisabeth.

"But if it were true that Garth--had shown cowardice, why was he not shot? They shoot men for cowardice"--grimly.

"There are many excuses to be made for him, Sara," replied Elisabeth gently.

"Excuses! For cowardice!" The low-spoken words were icy with a biting contempt. "I'm afraid I could not find them."

"The court-martial did, nevertheless. At the trial, the 'prisoner's friend'--in this instance, Garth's colonel, who was very fond of him and had always thought very highly of him--pleaded extenuating circumstances. Garth's youth, his previous good record, the conditions of the moment--the continuous mental and physical strain of the days preceding his sudden loss of nerve--all these things were urged by the 'prisoner's friend,' and the sentence was commuted to one of cashiering."

"It would have been better if he had been shot," said Sara dully. Then suddenly she clapped both hands to her mouth. "Ah--h! What am I saying? Garth! . . . Garth! . . ."

She stumbled to her feet, her white, ravaged face turned for a moment yearningly towards Far End, where it stood bathed in the mocking morning sunlight. Then she spun half-round, groping for support, and fell in a crumpled heap on the floor.

When Sara came to herself again, she was lying on the bed in Elisabeth's room at the hotel. Some one had drawn the blinds, shutting out the crude glare of the sunlight, and in the semi-darkness she could feel soft hands about her, bathing her face with something fragrantly cool and refreshing. She opened her eyes and looked up to find Elisabeth's face bent over her--unspeakably kind and tender, like that of some Madonna brooding above her child.

"Are you feeling better?" The sweet, familiar voice roused her to the realization of what had happened. It was the same voice that, before unconsciousness had wrapped her in its merciful oblivion, had been pouring into her ears an unbelievably hideous story--a nightmare tale of what had happened at some far distant Indian outpost.

The details of the story seemed to be all jumbled confusedly together in Sara's mind, but, as gradually full consciousness returned, they began to sort themselves and fall into their rightful places, and all at once, with a swift and horrible contraction of her heart, the truth knocked at the door of memory.

She struggled up on to her elbow, her eyes frantically appealing.

"Elisabeth, was it true? Was it--all true?"

In an instant Elisabeth's hand closed round hers.

"My dear, you must try and face it. And"--her voice shook a little--"you must try and forgive me for telling you. But I couldn't let you marry Garth Trent in ignorance, could I?"

"Then it is true? Garth was court-martialled and--and cashiered?" Sara sank back against her pillows. Still, deep within her, there flickered a faint spark of hope. Against all reason, against all common sense the faith that was within her fought against accepting the bitter knowledge that Garth was guilty of what was in her eyes the one unpardonable sin.

Unpardonable! The word started a new and overwhelming train of thought. She remembered that she had told Garth she did not care what sin he had been guilty of, had forced him to believe that nothing could make any difference to her love for him, to her willingness to become his wife, and share his burden. Yet now, now that the hidden thing in his life had been revealed to her, she found herself shrinking from it in utter loathing! Her promises of faith and loyalty were already crumbling under the strain of her knowledge of the truth.

She flinched from the recognition of the fact, seeking miserably to palliate and excuse it. When she had given Garth that impetuous assurance of her confidence, she had not, in her crudest imaginings, dreamed of anything so hideous and ignoble as the actual truth had proved to be. Vaguely, she had deemed him outcast for some big, reckless sin that by the splendour of its recklessness almost earned its own forgiveness.

And instead--*this*! This drab-hued, pitiful weakness for which she could find no pardon in her heart.

Through the turmoil of her thoughts she became conscious that Elisabeth was stooping over her, answering her wild incredulous questioning.

"Yes, it is true," she was saying steadily. "He was court-martialled and cashiered. But, if you still doubt it, ask him yourself, Sara."

Sara's hands clenched themselves. Her eyes were feverishly brilliant in her white, shrunken face.

"Yes, I'll ask him myself." She panted a little. "You must be wrong--there must be some horrible mistake somewhere. I've been mad--mad to believe it for a single moment." She slipped from the bed to her feet, and stood confronting Elisabeth with a kind of desperate defiance. "Do you hear what I say?" she said loudly. "I don't believe it. I will never believe it till Garth himself tells me that it is true."

"Oh, my dear"--Elisabeth shrank away a little, but her eyes were kind and infinitely pitying. Sara felt frightened of the pitying kindness in those eyes--its rejection of Garth's innocence was so much stronger than any asseveration of mere words. Vaguely she heard Elisabeth's patient voice: "I think you are right. Ask him yourself--but, Sara, he will not be able to deny it."

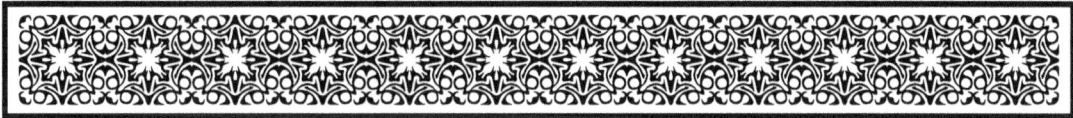

CHAPTER XXVIII
RED RUIN

"You sent for me, and I am here."

The brusque, curt speech sounded a knell to the faint hope which Sara had been tending whilst she waited for Garth's coming. His voice, the dogged expression of his face, the chill, brief manner, each held its grievous message for the woman who had learned to recognize the signs of mental stress in the man she loved.

"Yes, I sent for you," she said. "I--I--Garth, I have seen Elisabeth."

"Yes?" Just the one brief monosyllable in response, uttered with a slightly questioning inflection. Nothing more.

Sara twisted her hands together. There was something unapproachable about Garth as he stood there--quiet, inflexible, waiting to hear what she had to say to him.

With an effort she began again.

"She has told me of something--something that happened to you, in the past."

"Yes? Quite a great deal happened--in my past. What was it, in particular, that she told you?"

The mocking quality in his tones stung her into open accusation.

"She told me that you had been court-martialled and cashiered from the Army--for cowardice." The words came slowly, succinctly.

"Ah--h!" He drew his breath sharply, and a grey shadow seemed to spread itself over his face.

Sara waited--waited with an intensity of longing that was well-nigh unendurable--for either the indignant denial or the easy, mirthful scorn wherewith an innocent man might be expected to answer such a charge.

But there came neither of these. Only silence--an endless, agonizing silence, while Garth stood utterly motionless, looking at her, his face slowly greying.

It was impossible to interpret the expression of his eyes. There was neither anger, nor horror, nor pleading in their cool indomitable stare, but only a hard, bright impenetrability, shuttering the soul behind it from the aching gaze of the woman who waited.

In that silence, Sara's flickering hope that the accusation might prove false went out in blinding darkness. She *knew*, now--knew it as certainly as though Garth had answered her--that he was unable to deny it. Still, she would brace herself to hear it--to endure the ultimate anguish of words.

"Is it true?" she questioned him. "Is it true that you were--cashiered for cowardice?"

At last he spoke.

"Yes," he said. "It is true." His voice was altogether passionless, but something had come into his face, into his whole attitude, which denied the calm passivity of his reply. The soul of the man--a soul in ineffable extremity of suffering--was struggling for expression, striving against the rigid bonds of the motionless body in which his iron will constrained it.

Sara could sense it--a tormented flame shut in a casing of steel--and she was swept by a torrent of uttermost pity and compassion.

"Garth! Garth! But there must have been some explanation! . . . You weren't in your right senses at the moment. Ah! Tell me----" She broke off, her voice failing her, her arms outflung in a passion of entreaty.

As she leaned towards him, a tremor seemed to run through his entire body--the tremor of leaping muscles straining against the leash. His hands clenched slowly, the nails biting into the bruised flesh. Then he spoke, and his voice was ringing and assured--arrogantly so. The tortured soul within him had been beaten back once more into its prison-house.

"I was quite in my right senses--that night on the Frontier--never more so, believe me"--and his lips twisted in a curious, enigmatical smile. "And as far as explanations--excuses--are concerned, the court-martial made all that were possible. I--I was not shot, you see!"

There was something outrageous in the open derision of the last words. He flung them at her--as though taunting, gibing at the impulse to compassion which had swayed her, sending her tremulously towards him with imploring, outstretched hands.

"The quality of mercy was not strained in the least," he continued. "It fell around me like the proverbial gentle rain. I've quite a lot to be thankful for, don't you think?"--brutally.

"I--I don't know what to think!" she burst out. "That you--*you* should fall so low--so shamefully low."

"A man will do a good deal to preserve a whole skin, you know," he suggested hardily.

"Why do you speak like that?" she demanded in sharpened tones. "Do you want me to think worse of you than I do already?"

He took a step towards her and stood looking down at her with those bright, hard eyes.

"Yes, I do," he said decidedly. "I want you to think as badly of me as you possibly can. I want you to realize just what sort of a blackguard you had promised to marry, and when you've got that really clear in your mind, you'll be able to forget all about me and marry some cheerful young fool who hasn't been kicked out of the Army."

"As long as I live I shall never--be able--to forget that I loved--a coward." The words came haltingly from her lips. Then suddenly her shaking hands went up to her face, as though to shut him from her sight, and a dry, choking sob tore its way through her throat.

He made a swift stride towards her, then checked himself and stood motionless once more, in the utter quiescence of deliberately arrested movement. Only his hands, hanging stiffly at his sides, opened and shut convulsively, and his eyes should have been hidden. God never meant any man's eyes to wear that look of unspeakable torment.

When at last Sara withdrew her hands and looked at him again, his face was set like a mask, the lips drawn back a little from the teeth in a way that suggested a dumb animal in pain. But she was so hurt herself that she failed to recognize his infinitely greater hurt.

"I think--I think I hate you," she whispered.

His taut muscles seemed to relax.

"I hope you do," he said steadily. "It will be better so."

Something in the quiet acceptance of his tone moved her to a softer, more wistful emotion.

"If it had been anything--anything but that, Garth, I think I could have borne it."

There was a depth of appeal in the low-spoken words. But he ignored it, opposing a reckless indifference to her softened mood.

"Then it's just as well it wasn't 'anything but that.' Otherwise"--sardonically--"you might have felt constrained to abide by your rash promise to marry me."

His eyes flashed over her face, mocking, deriding. He had struck where she was most vulnerable, accusing where her innate honesty of soul admitted she had no defence, and she winced away from the speech almost as though it had been a blow upon her body.

It was true she had given her promise blindly, in ignorance of the facts, but that could not absolve her. It was not Garth who had forced the promise from her. It was she who had impetuously offered it, never conceiving such a possibility as that he might be guilty of the one sin for which, in her eyes, there could be no palliation.

"I know," she said unevenly. "I know. You have the right to remind me of my promise. I--I blame myself. It's horrible--to break one's word."

She was silent a moment, standing with bent head, her instinct to be fair, to play the game, combating the revulsion of feeling with which the knowledge of Garth's act of cowardice had filled her. When she looked up again there was a curious intensity in her expression, wanly decisive.

"Marriage for us--now--could never mean anything but misery." The effort in her voice was palpable. It was as though she were forcing herself to utter words from which her inmost being recoiled. "But I gave you my promise, and if--if you choose to hold me to it--"

"I don't choose!" He broke in harshly. "You may spare yourself any anxiety on that score. You are free--as free as though we had never met. I'm quite ready to bow to your decision that I'm not fit to marry you."

A little caught breath of unutterable relief fluttered between her lips. If he heard it, he made no sign.

"And now"--he turned as though to leave her--"I think that's all that need be said between us."

"It is not all"--in a low voice.

"What? Is there more still?" Again his voice held an insolent irony that lashed her like a whip. "Haven't you yet plumbed the full depths of my iniquity?"

"No. There is still one further thing. You said you loved me?"

"I did--I do still, if such as I may aspire to so lofty an emotion."

"It was a lie. Even"--her voice broke--"even in that you deceived me."

It seemed as though the tremulously uttered words pierced through his armour of sneering cynicism.

"No, in that, at least, I was honest with you." The bitter note of mockery that had rung through all his former speech was suddenly absent--muted, crushed out, and the quiet, steadfast utterance carried conviction even in Sara's reeling faith, shaking her to the very soul.

"But . . . Elisabeth? . . . You loved her once. And love--can't die, Garth."

"No," he said gravely. "Love can't die. But what I felt for Elisabeth was not love--not love as you and I understand it. It was the mad passion of a boy for an extraordinarily beautiful woman. She was an ideal--I invested her with all the qualities and spiritual graces that her beauty seemed to promise. But the Elisabeth I loved--didn't exist." He drew nearer her and, laying his hands on her shoulders, looked down at her with eyes that seemed to burn their way into the inmost depths of her being. "Whatever you may think of me, however low I may have fallen in your sight, believe me in this--that I have loved you and shall always love you, utterly and entirely, with my whole soul and body. It has not been an easy love--I fought against it with all my strength, knowing that it could only carry pain and suffering in its train for both of us. But it conquered me. And when you came to me that day, so courageously, holding out your hands, claiming the love that was unalterably yours--when you came to me like that, a little hurt and wounded because I had been so slow to speak my love--I yielded! Before God, Sara! I had been either more or less than a man had I resisted!"

The grip of his hands upon her shoulders tightened until it was actual pain, and she winced under it, shrinking away from him. He released her instantly, and she stood silently beside him, battling against the longing to respond to that deep, abiding love which neither now, nor ever again in life, would she be able to doubt.

That Garth loved her, wholly and completely, was an incontrovertible fact. She no longer felt the least lingering mistrust, nor even any prick of jealousy that he had once loved before. That boyish passion of the senses for Elisabeth was not comparable with this love which was the maturer growth of his manhood--a love that could only know fulfillment in the mystic union of body, soul, and spirit.

But this merely served to deepen the poignancy of the impending parting--for that she and Garth must part she recognized as inevitable.

Loving each other as men and women love but once in a lifetime, their love was destined to be for ever unconsummated. They were as irrevocably divided as though the seas of the entire world ran between them.

Wearily, in the flat, level tones of one who realizes that all hope is at an end, she stumbled through the few broken phrases which cancelled the whole happiness of life.

"It all seems so useless, doesn't it--your love and mine? . . . You've killed something that I felt for you--I don't quite know what to call it--respect, I suppose, only that sounds silly, because it was much more than that. I wish--I wish I didn't love you still. But perhaps that, too, will die in time. You see, you're not the man I thought I cared for. You're--you're something I'm *ashamed* to love--"

"That's enough!" he interrupted unsteadily. "Leave it at that. You won't beat it if you try till doomsday."

The pain in his voice pierced her to the heart, and she made an impulsive step towards him, shocked into quick remorse.

"Garth . . . I didn't mean it!"

"Oh yes, you meant it," he said. "Don't imagine that I'm blaming you. I'm not. You've found me out, that's all. And having discovered exactly how contemptible a person I am, you--very properly--send me away."

He turned on his heel, giving her no time to reply, and a moment later she was alone. Then came the clang of the house door as it closed behind him. To Sara, it sounded like the closing of a door between two worlds--between the glowing past and the grey and empty future.

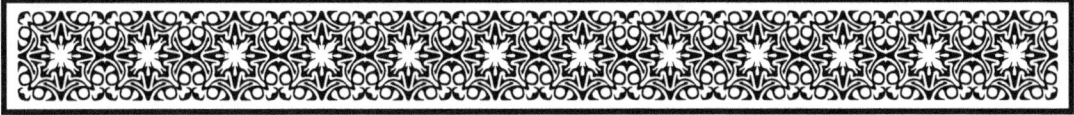

CHAPTER XXIX
DIVERS OPINIONS

The consternation created at Sunnyside by the breaking off of Sara's engagement had spent itself at last. Selwyn had said but little, only his saint's eyes held the wondering, hurt look that the inexplicable sins of humanity always had the power to bring into them. Characteristically, he hated the sin but overflowed in sympathy for the sinner.

"Poor devil!" he said, when the whole story of Trent's transgression and its consequences had been revealed to him. "What a ghastly stone to hang round a man's neck for the term of his natural life! If they'd shot him, it would have been more merciful! That would at least have limited the suffering," he went on, taking Sara's hand and holding it in his strong, kindly one a moment. "Poor little comrade! Oh, my dear"--as she shrank instinctively--"I'm not going to talk about it--I know you'd rather not. Condolence platitudes were never in my line. But my pal's troubles are mine--just as she once made mine hers."

Jane Crab's opinions were enunciated without fear or favour, and, in defiance of public opinion, she took her stand on the side of the sinner and maintained it unwaveringly.

"Well, Miss Sara," she affirmed, "unless you've proof as strong as 'Oly Writ, as they say, I'd believe naught against Mr. Trent. Bluff and 'ard he may be in 'is manner, but after the way he conducted himself the night Miss Molly ran away, I'll never think no ill of 'im, not if it was ever so!"

Sara smiled drearily.

"I wish I could feel as you do, Jane dear. But--Mrs. Durward *knows*."

"Mrs. Durward! Huh! One of them tigris women I calls 'er," retorted Jane, who had formed her opinion with lightning rapidity when Elisabeth made a farewell visit to Sunnyside before leaving Monkshaven. "Not but what you can't help liking her, neither," went on Jane judicially. "There's something good in the woman, for all she looks at you like a cat who thinks you're after stealing her kittens. But there! As the doctor--bless the man!--always says, there's good in everybody if so be you'll look for it. Only I'd as lief think that Mrs. Durward was somehow scared-like--too almighty scared to be her natchral self, savin' now and again when she forgets."

To Mrs. Selwyn, the breaking off of Sara's engagement, and the manner of it, signified very little. She watched the panorama of other people's lives unfold with considerably less sympathetic concern than that with which one follows the ups and downs that befall the characters in a cinema drama, since they were altogether outside the radius of that central topic of unfailing interest--herself.

The only way in which recent events impinged upon her life was in so far as the rupture of Sara's engagement would probably mean the indefinite prolongation of her stay at Sunnyside, which would otherwise have ended with her marriage. And this, from Mrs. Selwyn's egotistical point of view, was all to the good, since Sara had acquired a pleasant habit of making herself both useful and entertaining to the invalid.

Molly's emotions carried her to the other extreme of the compass. Since the night when she had realized that she had narrowly missed making entire shipwreck of her life, thanks to the evil genius of Lester Kent, her character seemed to have undergone a change--to have deepened and expanded. She was no longer so buoyantly superficial in her envisagement of life, and the big things reacted on her in a way which would previously have been impossible. Formerly, their significance would have passed her by, and she would have floated airily along, unconscious of their piercing reality.

Side by side with this increase of vision, there had developed a very deep and sincere affection for both Garth and Sara based, probably, in its inception, on her realization that whatever of good, whatever of happiness, life might hold for her, she would owe it fundamentally to the two who had so determinedly kept her heedless feet from straying into that desert from which there is no returning to the pleasant paths of righteousness. A censorious world sees carefully to that, for ever barring out the sinner--of the weaker sex--from inheriting the earth.

So that to this new and awakened Molly the abrupt termination of Sara's engagement came as something almost too overwhelming to be borne. She did not see how Sara *could* bear it, and to her youthful mind, mercifully unwitting that grief is one of the world's commonplaces, Sara was henceforth haloed with sorrow, set specially apart by the tragic circumstances which had enveloped her. Unconsciously she lowered her voice when speaking to her, infusing a certain specific sympathy into every small action she performed for her, shrank from troubling her in any way, and altogether, in her youth and inexperience, behaved rather as though she were in a house of mourning, where the candles yet burned in the chamber of death and the blinds shut out the light of day.

At last Sara rebelled, although compassionately aware of Molly's excellent intentions.

"Molly, my angel, if you persist in treating me as though I had just lost the whole of my relatives in an earthquake or a wreck at sea, I shall explode. I've had a bad knock, but I don't want it continually rubbing into me. The world will go on--even although my engagement is broken off. And *I'm* going on."

It was bravely spoken, and though Sara was inwardly conscious that in the last words the spirit, for the moment, outdistanced the flesh, it served to dissipate the rather strained atmosphere which had prevailed at Sunnyside since the rupture of her engagement had become common knowledge.

So, figuratively speaking, the blinds were drawn up and life resumed its normal aspect once again.

It had fallen to the lot of Audrey Maynard to carry the ill-tidings to Rose Cottage. Sara had asked her to acquaint their little circle with the altered condition of affairs, and Audrey had readily undertaken to perform this service, eager to do anything that might spare Sara some of the inevitable pinpricks which attend even the big tragedies of life.

"The whole affair is incomprehensible to me," said Audrey at last, as she rose preparatory to taking her departure. There seemed no object in lingering to discuss so painful a topic. "It's--oh! It's heart-breaking."

Miss Livinia departed hastily to do a little weep in the seclusion of her room upstairs. She hardly concerned herself with the enormity of Garth's offence. She was old, and she saw only romance shattered into fragments, youth despoiled of its heritage, love crucified. Moreover, the Lavender Lady had never been censorious.

"What is your opinion, Miles?" asked Audrey, when she had left the room.

Herrick had been rather silent, his brown eyes meditative. Now he looked up quickly.

"About the funking part of it? As I wasn't on the spot when the affair took place, I haven't the least right to venture an opinion."

Audrey looked puzzled.

"I don't see why not. You can't get behind the verdict of the court-martial."

"Trials have been known where justice went awry," said Miles quietly. "There was a trial where Pilate was judge."

"Do you mean to say you doubt the verdict?"--eagerly.

"No, I was not meaning quite that in this case. But, because the law says a man is a blackguard, when I'd stake my life he's nothing of the kind, it doesn't alter my opinion one hair's-breadth. The verdict may have been--probably, almost certainly, *was*--the only verdict that could be given to meet the facts of the case. But still, it is possible that it was not a just verdict--labelling as a coward for all time a man who may have had one bad moment when his nerves played him false. There are other men who have had their moment of funk, but, as the matter never came under the official eyes, they have made good since--ended up as V.C.'s, some of 'em. Facts are often very foolish things, to my mind. Motives, and circumstances, even conditions of physical health, are bound to play as big a part as facts, if you're going to administer pure justice. But the army can't consider the super-administration of justice"--smiling. "Discipline must be maintained and examples made. Only--sometimes--it's damn bad luck on the example."

It was an unusually long speech for Miles to have been guilty of, and Audrey stood looking at him in some surprise.

"Miles, you're rather a dear, you know. I believe you're almost as strongly on Garth's side as Jane Crab."

"Is Jane?" And Herrick smiled. "She's a good old sport then. Anyhow, I don't propose to add my quota to the bill Trent's got to pay, poor devil!"

Audrey's face softened as she turned to go.

"One can't help feeling pitifully sorry for him," she admitted. "To have had Sara--and then to have lost her!"

There was a whimsical light in Herrick's eyes as he answered her.

"But, at least," he said, "he *has* had her, if only for a few days."

Audrey paused with her hand upon the latch of the door.

"I imagine Garth--asked for what he wanted!" she observed, and vanished precipitately through the doorway.

"Audrey!" Miles started up, but, by the time he reached the house door, she was already disappearing through the gateway into the road and beyond pursuit.

"She must have *run*!" he commented ruefully to himself as he returned to the sitting-room.

This discovery seemed to afford him food for reflection. For a long time he sat very quietly in his chair, apparently arguing out with himself some knotty point.

Nor had his thoughts, at the moment, any connection with the recent discussion of Garth Trent's affairs. It was only after the Lavender Lady had returned, a little pink about the eyelids, that the recollection of the original object of Mrs. Maynard's visit recurred to him.

Simultaneously, his brows drew together in a sudden concentration of thought, and an inarticulate exclamation escaped him.

Miss Livinia looked up from the delicate piece of cobwebby lace she was finishing.

"What did you say, dear?" she asked absently.

"I didn't say anything," he smiled back at her. "I was thinking rather hard, that's all, and just remembered something I had forgotten."

The Lavender Lady looked a trifle mystified.

"I don't think I quite understand, Miles dear."

Herrick, on his way to the door, stooped to kiss her.

"Neither do I, Lavender Lady. That's just the devil of it," he answered cryptically.

He passed out of the room and upstairs, presently returning with a couple of letters, held together by an elastic band, in his hand.

They smelt musty as he unfolded them; evidently they had not seen the light of day for a good many years. But Miles seemed to find them of extraordinary interest, for he subjected the closely written sheets to a first, and second, and even a third perusal. Then he replaced the elastic band round them and shut them away in a drawer, locking the latter carefully.

A couple of days later, Garth Trent received a note from Herrick, asking him to come and see him.

"You haven't been near us for days," it ran. "Remember Mahomet and the mountain, and as I can't come to you, look me up."

The letter, in its quiet avoidance of any reference to recent events, was like cooling rain falling upon a parched and thirsty earth.

Since the history of the court-martial had become common property, Garth had been through hell. It was extraordinary how quickly the story had leaked out, passing from mouth to mouth until there was hardly a cottage in Monkshaven that was not in possession of it, with lurid and fictitious detail added thereto.

The chambermaid at the Cliff Hotel had been the primary source of information. From the further side of the connecting-door of an adjoining room, she had listened with interest to the conversation which had taken place between Elisabeth and Sara on the day following the Haven Woods picnic, and had proceeded to circulate the news with the avidity of her class. Nor had certain gossipy members of the picnic party refrained from canvassing threadbare the significance of the unfortunate scene which had taken place on that occasion--contributory evidence to the truth of the chambermaid's account of what she had overheard.

The whole town hummed with the tale, and Garth had not long been allowed to remain in ignorance of the fact. Anonymous letters reached him almost daily-- for it must be remembered that ten years of an aloof existence at Monkshaven had not endeared him to his neighbours. They had resented what they chose to consider his exclusiveness, and, now that it was so humiliatingly explained, the meaner spirits amongst them took this way of paying off old scores.

It was suggested by one of the anonymous writers that Trent's continued presence in the district was felt to be a blot on the fair fame of Monkshaven; and, by another, that should the rumours now flying hither and thither concerning the imminence of a European war materialize into fact, the French Foreign Legion offered opportunities for such as he.

Garth tore the letters into fragments, pitching them contemptuously into the waste-paper basket; but, nevertheless, they were like so many gnats buzzing about an open wound, adding to its torture.

Black Brady, with a lively recollection of the few days in gaol which Trent had procured him in recompense for his poaching proclivities, was loud in his denunciation.

"Retreated, they calls it," he observed, with fine scorn. "Runned away's the plain English of it."

And with this pronouncement all the loafers round the hotel garage cordially agreed, and, subsequently, black looks and muttered comments followed Garth's appearance in the streets.

To all of which Garth opposed a stony indifference--since, after all, these lesser things were of infinitely small moment to a man whose whole life was lying in ruins about him.

"It was good of you to ask me over," he told Herrick, as they shook hands. "Sure you're not afraid of contamination?"

"Quite sure," replied Miles, smiling serenely. "Besides, I had a particular reason for wishing to see you."

"What was that?"

Miles unlocked the drawer where he had laid aside the papers he had perused with so much interest two days ago, and, slipping them out of the elastic bands that held them, handed them to Trent.

"I'd like you to read those documents, if you will," he said.

There was a short silence while Trent's eyes travelled swiftly down the closely written sheets. When he looked up from their perusal his expression was perfectly blank. Miles could glean nothing from it.

"Well?" he said tentatively.

Garth quietly tendered him back the letters.

"You shouldn't believe everything you hear, Herrick," was all he vouchsafed.

"Then it isn't true?" asked Miles searchingly.

"It sounds improbable," replied Trent composedly.

Miles reflected a moment. Then, slowly replacing the papers within the elastic band, he remarked--

"I think I'll take Sara's opinion."

If he had desired to break down the other's guard of indifference, he succeeded beyond his wildest expectations.

Trent sprang to his feet, his hand outstretched as though to snatch the letters back again. His eyes blazed excitedly.

"No! No! You mustn't do that--you can't do that! It's----Oh! You won't understand--but those papers must be destroyed."

Herrick's fingers closed firmly round the papers in question, and he slipped them into the inside pocket of his coat.

"They certainly will not be destroyed," he replied. "I hold them in trust. But, tell me, why should I *not* show them to Sara? It seems to me the one obvious thing to do."

Trent shook his head.

"No. Believe me, it could do no good, and it might do an infinity of harm."

Herrick looked incredulous.

"I can't see that," he objected.

"It is so, nevertheless."

A silence fell between them.

"Then you mean," said Herrick, breaking it at last, "that I'm to hold my tongue?"

"Just that."

"It is very unfair."

"And if you published that information abroad, it's unfair to Tim. Have you thought of that? He, at least, is perfectly innocent."

"But, man, it's inconceivable--grotesque!"

"Not at all. I gave Elisabeth Durward my promise, and she has married and borne a son, trusting to that promise. My lips are closed--now and always."

"But mine are not."

"They will be, Miles, if I ask it. Don't you see, there's no going back for me now? I can't wipe out the past. I made a bad mistake--a mistake many a youngster similarly circumstanced might have made. And I've been paying for it ever since. I must go on paying to the end--it's my honour that's involved. That's why I ask you not to show those letters."

Miles looked unconvinced.

"I forged my own fetters, Herrick," continued Trent. "In a way, I'm responsible for Tim Durward's existence and I can't damn his chances at the outset. After all, he's at the beginning of things. I'm getting towards the end. At least"--wearily--"I hope so."

Herrick's quick glance took in the immense alteration the last few days had wrought in Trent's appearance. The man had aged visibly, and his face was worn and lined, the eyes burning feverishly in their sockets.

"You're good for another thirty or forty years, bar accidents," said Herrick at last, deliberately. "Are you going to make those years worse than worthless to you by this crazy decision?"

"I've no alternative. Good Lord, man!"--with savage irritability--"you don't suppose I'm enjoying it, do you? But I've **no way out**. I took a certain responsibility on myself--and I must see it through. I can't shirk it now, just because pay-day's come. I can do nothing except stick it out."

"And what about Sara?" said Herrick quietly. "Has she no claim to be considered?"

He almost flinched from the look of measureless anguish that leapt into the others man's eyes in response.

"For God's sake, man, leave Sara out of it!" Garth exclaimed thickly. "I've cursed myself enough for the suffering I've brought on her. I was a mad fool to let her know I cared. But I thought, as Garth Trent, that I had shut the door on the past. I ought to have known that the door of the past remains eternally ajar."

Miles nodded understandingly.

"I don't think you were to blame," he said. "It's Mrs. Durward who has pulled the door wide open. She's stolen your new life from you--the life you had built up. Trent, you owe that woman nothing! Let me show this letter, and the other that goes with it, to Sara!"

Trent shook his head in mute refusal.

"I can't," he said at last. "Elisabeth must be forgiven. The best woman in the world may lose all sense of right and wrong when it's a question of her child. But, even so, I can't consent to the making public of that letter." He rose and paced the room restlessly. "Man! Man!" he cried at last, coming to a halt in front of Herrick. "Can't you see--that woman trusted me with her whole life, and with the life of any child that she might bear, when she married on the strength of my promise. And I must keep faith with her. It's the one poor rag of honour left me, Herrick!"--with intense bitterness.

There was a long silence. Then, at last, Miles held out his hand.

"You've beaten me," he said sadly. "I won't destroy the letters. As I said, they are a trust. But the secret is safe with me, after this. You've tied my hands."

Trent smiled grimly.

"You'll get used to it," he commented. "Mine have been tied for three-and-twenty years--though even yet I don't wear my bonds with grace, precisely."

He had become once more the hermit of old acquaintance--sardonic, harsh, his emotions hidden beneath that curt indifference of manner with which those who knew him were painfully familiar.

The two men shook hands in silence, and a few minutes later, Herrick, left alone, replaced the letters in the drawer whence he had taken them, and, turning the key upon them, slipped it into his pocket.

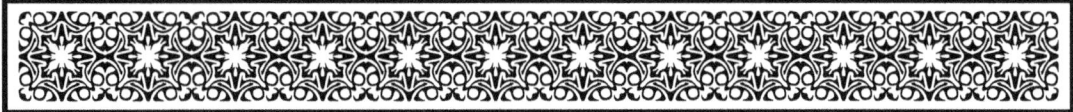

CHAPTER XXX
DEFEAT

In remote country districts that memorable Fourth of August, when England declared war on Germany, came and went unostentatiously.

People read the news a trifle breathlessly, reflected with a sigh of contentment on the invincible British Navy, and with a little gust of prideful triumph upon the Expeditionary force--ready to the last burnished button of each man's tunic--and proceeded quietly with their usual avocations.

Then came the soaring Bank Rate, and business men on holiday raced back to London to contend with the new financial conditions and assure their credit. That was all that happened--at first.

Few foresaw that the gaunt, grim Spectre of War had come to dwell in their very midst, nor that soon he would pass from house to house, palace and cottage alike, touching first this man, then that, on the shoulder, with the single word "Come!" on his lips, until gradually the nations, one by one, left their tasks of peace and rose and followed him.

Monkshaven, in common with other seaside towns, witnessed the sudden exodus of City men when the climbing Bank Rate sounded its alarm. Beyond that, the war, for the moment, reacted very little on its daily processes of life. There was no disorganization of amusements--tennis, boating, and bathing went on much as usual, and clever people, proud of their ability to add two and two together and make four of them, announced that it was all explained now why certain young officers in the neighbourhood had been hurriedly recalled a few days previously, and their leave cancelled.

Then came the black news of that long, desperate retreat from Mons, shaking the nation to its very soul, and in the wave of high courage and endeavour that swept responsively across the country, the smaller things began to fall into their little place.

To Sara, stricken by her own individual sorrow, the war came like a rushing, mighty wind, rousing her from the brooding, introspective habit which had laid hold of her and bracing her to take a fresh grip upon life. Its immense demands, the illimitable suffering it carried in its train, lifted her out of the contemplation of her own personal grief into a veritable passion of pity for the world agony beating up around her.

And, with Sara, to compassionate meant to succour. Nor did it require more than the first few weeks of war to demonstrate where such help as she was capable of giving was most sorely needed.

She had been through a course of First Aid and held her certificate, and, thanks to a year in France when she was seventeen--a much-grudged year, at the time, since it had separated her from her beloved Patrick--and to a natural facility for the language, inherited from her French forbears, she spoke French almost as fluently as she did English.

In France they were crying out for nurses, for at that period of the war there was work for any woman who had even a little knowledge plus the grit to face the horrors of those early days, and it was to France that Sara forthwith determined to go.

She had heard that an old friend of Patrick Lovell's, Lady Arronby by name, proposed equipping and taking over to France a party of nurses, and she promptly wrote to her, begging that she might be included in the little company.

Lady Arronby, who had been a sister at a London hospital before her marriage, recollected her old friend's ward very clearly. Sara rarely failed to make a definite impression, even upon people who only knew her slightly, and Lady Arronby, who had known her from her earliest days at Barrow, answered her letter without hesitation.

"I shall be delighted to have you with me," she had written. "Even though you are not a trained nurse, there's work out there for women of your caliber, my dear. So come. It will be a week or two yet before we have all our equipment, but I am pushing things on as fast as I can, so hold yourself in readiness to come at a day's notice."

Meanwhile, Sara's earliest personal encounter with the reality of the war came in a few hurried lines from Elisabeth telling her that Major Durward had rejoined the Army and would be going out to France almost immediately.

Sara thrilled, and with the thrill came the answering stab of the sword that was to pierce her again and again through the long months ahead. Garth Trent--the man she loved--could have no part nor lot in this splendid service of England's sons for England! The country wanted brave men now--not men who faltered when faltering meant failure and defeat.

She had not seen Garth since that day--a million years ago it seemed--when she had sent him from her, and he had gone, admitting the justice of her decision.

There was no getting behind that. She would have defied Elisabeth, defied a whole world of slanderous tongues, had they accused him, if he himself had denied the charge. But he had not been able to deny it. It was true--a deadly, official truth, tabulated somewhere in the records of her country, that the man she loved had been cashiered for cowardice.

The knowledge almost crushed her, and she sometimes wondered if there could be a keener suffering, in the whole gamut of human pain, than that which a woman bears whose high pride in her lover has been laid utterly in the dust.

The dread of danger, separation--even death itself--were not comparable with it. Sara envied the women whose men were killed in action. At least, they had a splendid memory to hold which nothing could ever soil or take away.

Sometimes her thoughts wandered fugitively to Tim. Surely here was his chance to break from the bondage his mother had imposed upon him! He had not written to her of late, but she felt convinced that she would have heard from Elisabeth had he volunteered. She was a little puzzled over his silence and inaction. He had seemed so keen last winter at Barrow, when together they had discussed this very subject of soldiering. Could it be that now, when the opportunity offered, Tim was--evading it? But the thought was dismissed almost as swiftly as it had arisen, and Sara blushed scarlet with shame that the bare suspicions should have crossed her mind, even for an instant, recognizing it as the outcrop of that bitter knowledge which had cut at the very roots of her belief in men's courage.

And there were men around her whose readiness to make the great sacrifice combated the poison of one man's failure. Daily she heard of this or that man whom she knew, either personally or by name, having volunteered and been accepted, and very often she had to listen to Miles Herrick's fierce rebellion against the fact that he was ineligible, and endeavour to console him.

But it was Audrey Maynard who plumbed the full depths of bitterness in Herrick's heart. She had been teaching him to knit, and he was floundering through the intricacies of turning his first heel when one day he surprised her by hurling the sock, needles and all, to the other end of the room.

"There's work for a man when his country's at war! My God! Audrey, I don't know how I'm going to bear it--to lie here on my couch, knitting--*knitting!*--when men are out there dying! Why won't they take a lame man? Can't a lame man fire a gun--and then die like the rest of 'em?"

Audrey looked at him pitifully.

"My dear, war takes only the best--the youngest and the fittest. But there's plenty of work for the women and men at home."

"For the women and crocks?" countered Miles bitterly.

She smiled at him suddenly.

"Yes--for the crocks, too."

He shook his head.

"No, Audrey, I'm an utterly useless person--a cumberer of the ground."

"Not in my eyes, Miles," she answered quietly.

He met her glance, and read, at last, what--as she told him later--he might have read there any time during the last six months, had he chosen to look for it.

"Do you mean that, Audrey?" he asked, suddenly gripping her hands hard. "All of it--all that it implies?"

She slipped to her knees beside his couch.

"Oh, my dear!" she said, between laughing and crying. "I've been meaning it--'all of it'--for ever so long. Only--only you won't ask me to marry you!"

"How can I? A lame man, and not even a rich one?"

"I believe," said Audrey composedly, "we've argued both those points before--from a strictly impersonal point of view! Couldn't you--couldn't you get over your objection to coming to live with me at Greenacres, dear?"

Audrey always declared, afterwards, that it had required the most blatant encouragement on her part to induce Miles to propose to her, and that, but for the war--which convinced him that he was of no use to any one else--he never would have done so.

Presumably she was able to supply the requisite stimulus, for when the Lavender Lady joined them later on in the afternoon, she found herself called upon to perform that function of sheer delight to every old maid of the right sort--namely, to bestow her blessing on a pair of newly betrothed lovers.

Sara received the news the next morning, and though naturally, by contrast, it seemed to add a keener edge to her own grief, she was still able to rejoice wholeheartedly over this little harvesting of joy which her two friends had snatched from amid the world's dreadful harvesting of pain and sorrow.

By the same post as the radiant letters from Miles and Audrey came one from Elisabeth Durward. She wrote distractedly.

"Tim is determined to volunteer," ran her letter. "I can't let him go, Sara. He is my only son, and I don't see why he should be claimed from me by this horrible war. I have persuaded him to wait until he has seen you. That is all he will consent to. So will you come and do what you can to dissuade him? There is a cord by which you could hold him if you would."

A transient smile crossed Sara's face as she pictured Tim gravely consenting to await her opinion on the matter. He knew--none better!--what it would be, and, without doubt, he had merely agreed to the suggestion in the hope that her presence might ease the strain and serve to comfort his mother a little.

Sara telegraphed that she would come to Barrow Court the following day, and, on her arrival, found Tim waiting for her at the station in his two-seater.

"Well," he said with a grin, as the little car slid away along the familiar road. "Have you come to persuade me to be a good boy and stay at home, Sara?"

"You know I've not," she replied, smiling. "I'm gong to talk sense to Elisabeth. Oh! Tim boy, how I envy you! It's splendid to be a man these days."

He nodded silently, but she could read in his expression the tranquil satisfaction that his decision had brought. She had seen the same look on other men's faces, when, after a long struggle with the woman-love that could not help but long to hold them back, the final decision had been taken.

Arrived at the lodge gates, Tim handed over the car to the chauffeur who met them there, evidently by arrangement.

"I thought we'd walk across the park," he suggested.

Sara acquiesced delightedly. There was a tender, reminiscent pleasure in strolling along the winding paths that had once been so happily familiar, and, hardly conscious of the sudden silence which had fallen upon her companion, her thoughts slipped back to the old days at Barrow when she had wandered, with Patrick beside her in his wheeled chair, along these selfsame paths.

With a little thrill, half pain, half pleasure, she noted each well-remembered landmark. There was the arbour where they used to shelter from a shower, built with sloped boards at its entrance so that Patrick's chair could easily be wheeled into it; now they were passing the horse-chestnut tree which she herself had planted years ago--with the head gardener's assistance!--in place of one that had been struck by lightning. It had grown into a sturdy young sapling by this time. Here was the Queen's Bench--an old stone seat where Queen Elisabeth was supposed to have once sat and rested for a few minutes when paying a visit to Barrow Court. Sara reflected, with a smile, that if history speaks truly, the Virgin Queen must have spent quite a considerable portion of her time in visiting the houses of her subjects! And here--

"Sara!" Tim's voice broke suddenly across the recollections that were thronging into her mind. There was a curious intent quality in his tone that arrested her attention, filling her with a nervous foreboding of what he had to say.

"Sara, you know, of course, as well as I do, that I am going to volunteer. I let mother send for you, because--well, because I thought you would make it a little easier for her, for one thing. But I had another reason."

"Had you?" Sara spoke mechanically. They had paused beside the Queen's Bench, and half-unconsciously she laid her ungloved hand caressingly on the seat's high back. The stone struck cold against the warmth of her flesh.

"Yes." Tim was speaking again, still in that oddly direct manner. "I want to ask you--now, before I go to France--whether there will ever be any chance for me?"

Sara turned her eyes to his face.

"You mean----"

"I mean that I'm asking you once again if you will marry me? If you will--if I can go away leaving *my wife* in England, I shall have so much the more to fight for. But if you can't give me the answer I wish--well"--with a curious little smile--"it will make death easier, should it come--that's all."

The quiet, grave directness of the speech was very unlike the old, impetuous Tim of former days. It brought with it to Sara's mind a definite recognition of the fact that the man had replaced the boy.

"No, Tim," she responded quietly. "I made one mistake--in promising to marry you when I loved another man. I won't repeat it."

"But"--Tim's face expressed sheer wonder and amazement--"you don't still care for Garth Trent--for that blackguard? Oh!" remorsefully, as he saw her wince--"forgive me, Sara, but this war makes one feel even more bitterly about such a thing than one would in normal times."

"I know--I understand," she replied quietly. "I'm--ashamed of loving him." She turned her head restlessly aside. "But, don't you see, love can't be made and unmade to order. It just *happens*. And it's happened to me. In the circumstances, I can't say I like it. But there it is. I do love Garth--and I can't *unlove* him. At least, not yet."

"But some day, Sara, some day?" he urged.

She shook her head.

"I shall never marry anybody now, Tim. If--if ever I 'get over' this fool feeling for Garth, I know how it would leave me. I shall be quite cold and hard inside--like that stone"--pointing to the Queen's Bench. "I wish--I wish I had reached that stage now."

Silently Tim held out his hand, and she laid hers within it, meeting his grave eyes.

"I won't ever bother you again," he said, at last, quietly. "I think I understand, Sara, and--and, old girl, I'm awfully sorry. I wish I could have saved you--that."

He stooped his head and kissed her--frankly, as a big brother might, and Sara, recognizing that henceforth she would find in him only the good comrade of earlier days, kissed him back.

"Thank you, Tim," she said. "I knew you would understand. And, please, we won't ever speak of it again."

"No, we won't speak of it again," he answered.

He tucked his arm under hers, and they walked on together in the direction of the house.

"And now," she said, "let's go to Elisabeth and break it to her that we are--

both--going out to France as soon as we can get there."

He turned to look at her.

"You?" he exclaimed. "You going out? What do you mean?"

"I'm going with Lady Arronby. I want to go--badly. I want to be in the heart of things. You don't suppose"--with a rather shaky little laugh--"that I can stay quietly at home in England--and knit, do you?"

"No, I suppose *you* couldn't. But I don't half like it. The women who go--out there--have got to face things. I shan't like to think of you running risks--"

She laughed outright.

"Tim, if you talk nonsense of that kind, I'll revenge myself by urging Elisabeth to keep you at home," she declared. "Oh! Tim boy, can't you see that just now I must have something to do--something that will fill up every moment--and keep me from thinking!"

Tim heard the cry that underlay the words. There was no misunderstanding it. He squeezed her arm and nodded.

"All right, old thing, I won't try to dissuade you. I can guess a little of how you're feeling."

Sara's interview with Elisabeth was very different from anything she had expected. She had anticipated passionate reproaches, tears even, for an attractive women who has been consistently spoiled by her menkind is, of all her sex, the least prepared to bow to the force of circumstances.

But there was none of these things. It almost seemed as though in that first searching glance of hers, which flashed from Sara's face to the well-beloved one of her son, Elisabeth had recognized and accepted that, in the short space of time since these two had met, the decision concerning Tim's future had been taken out of her hands.

It was only when, in the course of their long, intimate talk together, she had drawn from Sara the acknowledgment that she had once again refused to be Tim's wife, that her control wavered.

"But, Sara, surely--surely you can't still have any thought of marrying Garth Trent?" There was a hint of something like terror in her voice.

"No," Sara responded wearily. "No, I shall never marry--Garth Trent."

"Then why won't you--why can't you--"

"Marry Tim?"--quietly. "Because, although I shall never marry Garth now, I haven't stopped loving him."

"Do you mean that you can still care for him--now that you know what kind of man he is?"

"Oh! Good Heavens, Elisabeth!"--the irritation born of frayed nerves hardened Sara's voice so that it was almost unrecognizable--"you can't turn love on and off as you would a tap! I shall never marry *anybody* now. Tim understands that, and--you must understand it, too."

There was no mistaking her passionate sincerity. The truth--that Sara would never, as long as she lived, put another in the place Garth Trent had held--seemed borne in upon Elisabeth that moment.

With a strangled cry she sank back into her chair, and her eyes, fixed on Sara's small, stern-set face, held a strange, beaten look. As she sat there, her hands gripping the chair-arms, there was something about her whole attitude that suggested defeat.

"So it's all been useless--quite useless!" she muttered in a queer, whispering voice.

She was not looking at Sara now. Her vision was turned inward, and she seemed to be utterly oblivious of the other's presence. "Useless!" she repeated, still in that strange, whispering tone.

"What has been useless?" asked Sara curiously.

Elisabeth started, and stared at her for a moment in a vacant fashion. Then, all at once, her mind seemed to come back to the present, and simultaneously the familiar watchful look sprang into her eyes. Sara was oddly conscious of being reminded of a sentry who has momentarily slept at his post, and then, awakening suddenly, feverishly resumed his vigilance.

"What was I saying?" Elisabeth brushed her hand distressfully across her forehead.

"You said that it had all been useless," repeated Sara. "What did you mean?"

Elisabeth paused a moment before replying.

"I meant that all my hopes were useless," she explained at last. "The hopes I had that some day you would be Tim's wife."

"Yes, they're quite useless--if that is what you meant," replied Sara. But there was a perplexed expression in her eyes. She had a feeling that Elisabeth was not be-ing quite frank with her--that that whispered confession of failure signified some-thing other than the simple interpretations vouchsafed.

The thing worried her a little, nagging at the back of her mind with the perti-nacity common to any little unexplained incident that has caught one's attention. But, in the course of a few days, the manifold happenings of daily life drove it out of her thoughts, not to recur until many months had passed and other issues paved the way for its resurgence.

Sara remained at Barrow until Tim had volunteered and been accepted, and the settlement of her own immediate plans synchronizing with this last event, it came about that it was only two hours after Tim's departure that she, too, bade farewell to Elisabeth, in order to join up in London with Lady Arronby's party.

Elisabeth stood at the head of the great flight of granite steps at Barrow and waved her hand as the car bore Sara swiftly away, and across the latter's mind flashed the memory of that day, nearly a year ago, when she herself had stood in the same place, waiting to welcome Elisabeth to her new home.

The contrast between then and now struck her poignantly. She recalled Elisa-beth as she had been that day--gracious, smiling, queening it delightfully over her two big men, husband and son, who openly worshipped her. Now, there remained only a great empty house, and that solitary figure on the doorstep, standing there with white face and lips that smiled perfunctorily.

Elisabeth turned slowly back into the house as the car disappeared round the curve of the drive. For her, the moment was doubly bitter. One by one, husband, son, and the woman whom she had ardently longed to see that son's wife, had been claimed from her by the pitiless demands of the madness men call War.

But there was still more for her to face. There was the utter downfall of all her hopes, the defeat of all her purposes. She had striven with the whole force that was in her to assure Tim's happiness. To compass this, she had torn down the curtain of the past, proclaiming a man's shame and hurling headlong into the dust the new life he had built up for himself, and with it had gone a woman's faith, and trust, and happiness.

And it had all been so futile! Two lives ruined, and the purchase price paid in tears of blood; and, after all, Tim's happiness was as utterly remote and beyond attainment as though no torrent of disaster had been let loose to further it! Elisabeth had bartered her soul in vain.

In the solitude which was all the war had left her, she recognized this, and, since she was normally a woman of kind and generous impulses, she suffered in the realization of the spoiled and mutilated lives for which she was responsible.

Not that she would have acted differently were the same choice presented to her again. She did not **want** to hurt people, but the primitive maternal instinct, which was the pivot of her being, blinded her to the claims of others if those claims reacted adversely on her son.

Only now, in the bitterness of defeat, as she looked back upon her midnight interview with Garth Trent, she was conscious of a sick repugnance. It had not been a pleasant thing, that thrusting of a knife into an old wound. This, too, she had done for Tim's sake. The pity of it was that Garth had suffered needlessly--uselessly!

She had thought the issue of events hung solely betwixt him and her son, and, with her mind concentrated on this idea, she had overlooked the possibility of any other outcome. But the acceptance of an unexpected sequence had been forced upon her--Sara would never marry any one now! Elisabeth recognized that all her efforts had been in vain.

And the supreme bitterness, from which all that was honest and upright within her shrank with inward shame and self-loathing, lay in the fact that she, above all others, owed Garth Trent--that which he had begged of her in vain--the tribute of silence concerning the past.

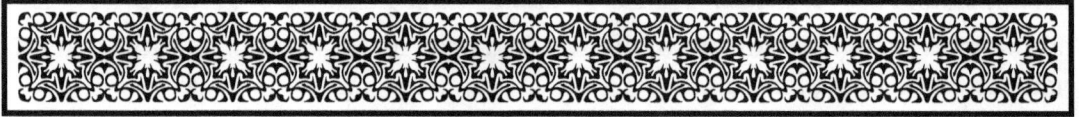

CHAPTER XXXI
THE FURNACE

As Sara took her seat on board the train for Monkshaven, she was conscious of that strange little thrill of the wanderer returned which is the common possession of the explorer and of the school-girl at their first sight of the old familiar scenes from which they have been exiled.

She could hardly believe that barely a year had elapsed since she had quitted Monkshaven. So many things had happened--so many changes taken place. Audrey had been transformed into Mrs. Herrick; Tim had been given a commission; and Molly, the one-time butterfly, was now become a working-bee--a member of the V.A.D. and working daily at Oldhampton Hospital. Sara could scarcely picture such a metamorphosis!

The worst news had been that of Major Durward's death--he had been killed in action, gallantly leading his men, in the early part of the year. Elisabeth had written to Sara at the time--a wonderfully brave, simple letter, facing her loss with a fortitude which Sara, remembering her adoration for her husband and her curious antipathy to soldiering as a profession, had not dared to anticipate. There was something rather splendid about her quiet acceptance of it. It was Elisabeth at her best--humanly hurt and broken, but almost heroic in her endurance now that the blow had actually fallen. And Sara prayed that no further sacrifice might be demanded from her--prayed that Tim might come through safely. For herself, she mourned Geoffrey Durward as one good comrade does another. She knew that his death would leave a big gap in the ranks of those she counted friends.

It had been a wonderful year--that year which she had passed in France--wonderful in its histories of tragedy and self-sacrifice, and in its revelation both of the brutality and of the infinite fineness of humanity. Few could have passed through such an experience and remained unchanged, certainly no one as acutely sentient and receptive as Sara.

She felt as though she had been pitchforked into a vast melting-pot, where the cast-iron generalizations and traditions which most people consider their opinions grew flexible and fluid in the scorching heat of the furnace, assimilating so much of the other ingredients in the cauldron that they could never reassume their former unqualified and rigid state.

And now that year of crowded life and ardent service was over, and she was side-tracked by medical orders for an indefinite period.

"Go back to England," her doctor had told her, "to the quietest corner in the country you can find--and try to forget that there *is* a war!"

This thin, eager-faced young woman, of whom every one on the hospital staff spoke in such glowing terms, interested him enormously. He could see that her year's work had taken out of her about double what it would have taken out of any one less sensitively alive, and he made a shrewd guess that something over and above the mere hard work accounted for that curiously fine-drawn look which he had observed in her.

During a hastily snatched meal, before the advent of another batch of casualties, he had sounded Lady Arronby on the subject. The latter shook her head.

"I can tell you very little. I believe there was a bad love-affair just before the war. All I know is that she was engaged and that the engagement was broken off very suddenly."

"Humph! And she's been living on her reserves ever since. Pack her off to England--and do it quick."

So October found Sara back in England once again, and as the train steamed into Monkshaven station, and her eager gaze fell on the little group of people on the platform, waiting to welcome her return, she felt a sudden rush of tears to her eyes.

She winked them away, and leaned out of the window. They were all there--big Dick Selwyn, and Molly, looking like a masquerading Venus in her V.A.D. uniform, the Lavender Lady and Miles, and--radiant and well-turned-out as ever--Mile's wife.

The Herrick's wedding had taken place very unobtrusively. About a month after Sara had crossed to France, Miles and Audrey had walked quietly into church one morning at nine o'clock and got married.

Monkshaven had been frankly disappointed. The gossips, who had so frequently partaken of Audrey's hospitality and then discussed her acrimoniously, had counted upon the lavish entertainment with which, even in war-time, the wedding of a millionaire's widow might be expected to be celebrated.

Instead of which, there had been this "hole-and-corner" sort of marriage, as the disappointed femininity of Monkshaven chose to call it, and, after a very brief honeymoon, Miles and Audrey had returned and thrown themselves heart and soul into the work of organizing and equipping a convalescent hospital for officers, of which Audrey had undertaken to bear the entire cost.

Henceforth the mouths of Audrey's detractors were closed. She was no longer "that shocking little widow with the dyed hair," but a woman who had married into a branch of one of the oldest families in the county, and whose immense private fortune had enabled her to give substantial help to her country in its need.

"I think it's simply splendid of you, Audrey," declared Sara warmly, as they were all partaking of tea at Greenacres, whither Audrey's car had borne them from the station.

Audrey laughed.

"My dear, what else could I do with my money? I've got such a sickening lot of it, you see! Besides"--with a bantering glance at her husband--"I think it was only the prospect of being of some use at my hospital which induced Miles to marry me! He's my private secretary, you know, and boss of the commissariat department."

Miles saluted.

"Quartermaster, at your service, miss," he said cheerfully, adding with a chuckle: "I saw my chance of getting a job if I married Audrey, so of course I took it."

He was looking amazingly well. The fact of being of some use in the world had acted upon him like a tonic, and there was no misinterpreting the glance of complete and happy understanding that passed between him and his wife.

Glad as she was to see it, it served to remind Sara painfully of all that she had missed, to stir anew the aching longing for Garth Trent, which, though struggled against, and beaten down, and sometimes temporarily crowded out by the thousand claims of each day's labour, had been with her all through the long months of her absence from Monkshaven.

It was this which had worn her so fine, not the hard physical work that she had been doing. Always slender, and built on racing lines, there was something almost ethereal about her now, and her sombre eyes looked nearly double their size in her small face of which the contour was so painfully distinct. Yet she was as vivid and alive as ever; she seemed to diffuse, as it were, a kind of spiritual brilliance.

"She makes one think of a flame," Audrey told her husband when they were alone once more. "There is something so *vital* about her, in spite of that curiously frail look she has."

Miles nodded.

"She's burning herself out," he said briefly.

Audrey looked startled.

"What do you mean, Miles?"

"Good Heavens! I should think it's self-evident. She's exactly as much in love with Trent as she was a year ago, and she's fighting against it every hour of her life. And the strain's breaking her."

"Can't we do something to help?" Audrey put her question with a helpless consciousness of its futility.

Herrick's eyes kindled.

"Nothing," he answered with quiet decision. "Every one must work out his own salvation--if it's to be a salvation worth having."

Herrick had delved to the root of the matter when he had declared that Sara was exactly as much in love as she had been a year ago.

She had realized this for herself, and it had converted life into an endless conflict between her love for Garth and her shamed sense of his unworthiness. And now, her return to Monkshaven, to its familiar, memory-haunted scenes, had quickened the struggle into new vitality.

With the broadened outlook born of her recent experiences, she began to ask herself whether a man need be condemned, utterly and for ever, for a momentary loss of nerve--even Elisabeth had admitted that it was probably no more than that! And then, conversely, her fierce detestation of that particular form of weakness, inculcated in her from her childhood by Patrick Lovell, would spring up protestingly, and she would shrink with loathing from the thought that she had given her love to a man who had been convicted of that very thing.

Nor was the attitude he had assumed in regard to the war calculated to placate her. She had learned from Molly that he had abstained from taking up any form of war-work whatsoever. He appeared to be utterly indifferent to the need of the moment, and the whole of Monkshaven buzzed with patriotic disapprobation of his conduct. There were few idle hands there now. A big munitions factory had been established at Oldhampton, and its demands, added to the necessities of the hospital, left no loophole of excuse for slackers.

Sara reflected bitterly that the sole courage of which Garth seemed possessed was a kind of cold, moral courage--brazen-facedness, the townspeople termed it--which enabled him to refuse doggedly to be driven out of Monkshaven, even though the whole weight of public opinion was dead against him.

And then the recollection of that day on Devil's Hood Island, when he had deliberately risked his life to save her reputation, would return to her with overwhelming force--mocking the verdict of the court-martial, repudiating the condemnation which had made her thrust him out of her life.

So the pendulum swung, this way and that, lacerating her heart each time it swept forward or back. But the blind agony of her recoil, when she had first learned the story of that tragic happening on the Indian frontier, was passed.

Then, overmastered by the horror of the thing, she had flung violently away from Garth, feeling herself soiled and dishonoured by the mere fact of her love for him, too revolted to contemplate anything other than the severance of the tie between them as swiftly as possible.

Now, with the widened sympathies and understanding which the past year of intimacy with human nature at its strongest, and at its weakest, had brought her, new thoughts and new possibilities were awaking within her.

The furnace--that fiercely burning furnace of life at its intensest--had done its work.

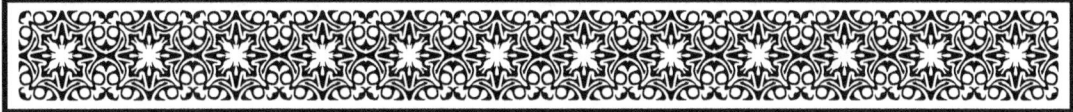

CHAPTER XXXII
ON CRABTREE MOOR

"Tim is wounded, and has been recommended for the Military Cross."

Sara made the double announcement quite calmly. The two things so often went together--it was the grey and gold warp and waft of war with which people had long since grown pathetically familiar.

"How splendid!" Molly enthused with sparkling eyes, adding quickly, "I hope he's not very badly wounded?"

"Elisabeth doesn't give any particulars in her letter. I can't understand her," Sara continued, her brows contracting in a puzzled fashion. "She seems so calm about it. She has always hated the idea of Tim's soldiering, yet now, although she's lost her husband and her son is wounded, she's taking it finely."

Selwyn looked up from filling his pipe.

"She's answering to the call--like every one else," he observed quietly.

"No." Sara shook her head. "I don't feel as though it were that. It's something more individual. Perhaps"--thoughtfully--"it's pride of a kind. The sort of impression I have is that she's so proud--so proud of Geoffrey's fine death, and of Tim's winning the Military Cross, that it has compensated in some way."

"The war's full of surprises," remarked Molly reflectively. "I never was so astonished in my life as when I found that Lester Kent's wife believed him to be a model of all the virtues! I wrote and told you--didn't I, Sara?--that he was sent to Oldhampton Hospital? He got smashed up, driving a motor ambulance, you know."

"Yes, you wrote and said that he died in hospital."

"Well, his wife came to see him, with her little boy. She was the sweetest thing, and so plucky. 'My dear,' she said to me, after it was all over, 'I hope you'll find a husband as dear and good. He was so loyal and true--and now that he's gone, I shall always have that to remember!'" Molly's eyes had grown very big and bright. "Oh! Sara," she went on, catching her breath a little, "supposing you hadn't brought me home--that night, she would have had no beautiful memory to help her now."

"And yet the memory is an utterly false one--though I suppose it will help her just the same! It's knowing the truth that hurts, sometimes." And Sara's lips twisted a little. "What a droll world it is--of shame and truth all mixed up--the ugly and the beautiful all lumped together!"

"And just now," put in Selwyn quietly, "it's so full of beauty."

"Beauty?" exclaimed both girls blankly.

Selwyn nodded, his eyes luminous.

"Isn't heroism beautiful--and self-sacrifice?" he said. "And this war's full of it. Sometimes, when I read the newspapers, I think God Himself must be surprised at the splendid things the men He made have done."

Sara turned away, swept by the recollection of one man she knew who had nothing splendid, nothing glorious, to his credit. Almost invariably, any discussion of the war ended by hurting her horribly.

"I'll take that basket of flowers across to the 'Convalescent' now, I think," she said, rising abruptly from her seat by the fire.

Selwyn nodded, mentally anathematizing himself for having driven her thoughts inward, and Molly, who had developed amazingly of late, tactfully refrained from offering to accompany her.

The Convalescent Hospital, situated on the crest of a hill above the town, was a huge mansion which had been originally built by a millionaire named Rattray, who, coming afterwards to financial grief, had found himself too poor to live in it when it was completed. It had been frankly impossible as a dwelling for any one less richly dowered with this world's goods, and, in consequence, when the place was thrown on the market, no purchaser would be found for it--since Monkshaven offered no attraction to millionaires in general.

Since then it had been known as Rattray's Folly, and it was not until Audrey cast covetous eyes upon it for her convalescent soldiers that the "Folly" had served any purpose other than that of a warning to people not to purchase boots too big for them.

A short cut from Sunnyside to the hospital lay through Crabtree Moor, and as Sara took her way across the rough strip of moorland, dotted with clumps of gorse and heather, her thoughts flew back to that day when she and Garth had encountered Black Brady there, and to the ridiculous quarrel which had ensued in consequence of Garth's refusal to condone the man's offence. For days they had not spoken to each other.

Looking backward, how utterly insignificant seemed that petty disagreement now! Had she but known the bitter separation that must come, she would have let no trifling difference, such as this had been, rob her of a single precious moment of their friendship.

She wondered if she and Garth would ever meet again. She had been back in Monkshaven for some weeks now, but he had studiously avoided meeting her, shutting himself up within the solitude of Far End.

And then, with her thoughts still centred round the man she loved, she lifted her eyes and saw him standing quite close to her. He was leaning against a gate which gave egress from the moor into an adjacent pasture field towards which her steps were bent. His arms, loosely folded, rested upon the top of the gate, and he was looking away from her towards the distant vista of sea and cliff. Evidently he had not heard her light footsteps on the springy turf, for he made no movement, but remained absorbed in his thoughts, unconscious of her presence.

Sara halted as though transfixed. For an instant the whole world seemed to rock, and a black mist rose up in front of her, blotting out that solitary figure at the gateway. Her heart beat in great, suffocating throbs, and her throat ached unbearably, as if a hand had closed upon it and were gripping it so tightly that she could not breathe. Then her senses steadied, and her gaze leapt to the face outlined in profile against the cold background of the winter sky.

Her searching eyes, poignantly observant, sensed a subtle difference in it--or, perhaps, less actually a difference than a certain emphasizing of what had been before only latent and foreshadowed. The lean face was still leaner than she had known it, and there were deep lines about the mouth--graven. And the mouth itself held something sternly sweet and austere about the manner of its closing--a severity of self-discipline which one might look to see on the lips of a man who has made the supreme sacrifice of his own will, bludgeoning his desires into submission in response to some finely conceived impulse.

The recognition of this, of the something fine and splendid that had stamped itself on Garth's features, came to Sara in a sudden blazoning flash of recognition. This was not--could not be the face of a weak man or a coward! And for one transcendent moment of glorious belief sheer happiness overwhelmed her.

But, in the same instant, the damning facts stormed up at her--the verdict of the court-martial, the details Elisabeth had supplied, above all, Garth's own inability to deny the charge--and the light of momentary ecstasy flared and went out in darkness.

An inarticulate sound escaped her, forced from her lips by the pang of that sudden frustration of leaping hope, and, hearing it, Garth turned and saw her.

"Sara!" The name rushed from his lips, shaken with a tumult of emotion. And then he was silent, staring at her across the little space that separated them, his hand gripping the topmost bar of the gate as though for actual physical support.

The calm of his face, that lofty serenity which had been impressed upon it, was suddenly all broken up.

"Sara!" he repeated, a ring of incredulity in his tones.

"Yes," she said flatly. "I've come back."

She moved towards him, trying to control the trembling that had seized her limbs.

"I--I've just come back from France," she added, making a lame attempt to speak conventionally.

It was an effort to hold out her hand, and, when his closed around it, she felt her whole body thrill at his touch, just as it had been wont to thrill in those few, short, golden days when their mutual happiness had been undarkened by any shadow from the past. Swiftly, as though all at once afraid, she snatched her hand from his clasp.

"What have you been doing in France?" he asked.

"Nursing," she answered briefly. "Did you think I could stay here and do-- nothing, at such a time as this?"

There was accusation in her tone, but if he felt that her speech reflected in any way upon himself, he showed no sign of it. His eyes were roving over her, marking the changes wrought in the year that had passed since they had met--the sharpened contour of her face, the too slender body, the white fragility of the bare hand which grasped the handle of the basket she was carrying.

"You are looking very ill," he said, at last, abruptly.

"I'm not ill," she replied indifferently. "Only a bit over-tired. As soon as I have had a thorough rest I am going back to France."

"You won't go back there again?" he exclaimed sharply. "You're not fit for such work!"

"Certainly I shall go back--as soon as ever Dr. Selwyn will let me. It's little enough to do for the men who are giving--everything!" Suddenly, the pent-up indignation within her broke bounds. "Garth, how can you stay here when men are fighting, dying--out there?" Her voice vibrated with the sense of personal shame which his apathy inspired in her. "Oh!"--as though she feared he might wound her yet further by advancing the obvious excuse--"I know you're past military age. But other men--older men than you--have gone. I know a man of fifty who bluffed and got in! There are heaps of back doors into the Army these days."

"And there's a back door out of it--the one through which I was kicked out!" he retorted, his mouth setting itself in the familiar bitter lines.

The scoffing defiance of his attitude baffled her.

"Don't you want to help your country?" she pleaded. It was horrible to her that he should stand aside--inexplicable except in terms of that wretched business on the Indian Frontier, in the hideous truth of which only his own acknowledgment had compelled her to believe.

He looked at her with hard, indifferent eyes.

"My country made me an outcast," he replied. "I'll remain such."

Somehow, even in her shamed bewilderment and anger, she sensed the hurt that lay behind the curt speech.

"Men who have been cashiered, men who are too old--they're all going back," she urged tremulously, snatching at any weapon that suggested itself.

He shrugged his shoulders.

"Let them!"

She stared at him in silence. She felt exactly as though she had been beating against a closed door. With a gesture of hopelessness she turned away, recognizing the futility of pleading with him further.

"One moment"--he stepped in front of her, barring her path. "I want an answer to a question before you go."

There was something of his old arrogance in the demand--the familiar, domi-nating quality which had always swayed her. Despite herself, she yielded to it now.

"Well?" she said unwillingly. "What is it you wish to know?"

"I want to know if you are engaged to Tim Durward."

For an instant the colour rushed into Sara's white face; then it ebbed away, leaving it paler than before.

"No," she said quietly. "I am not." She lifted her eyes, accusing, passionately reproachful, to his. "How could you--even ask me that? Did you ever believe I loved you?" she went on fiercely. "And if I did--could I care for any one else?"

A look of triumph leapt into his eyes.

"You care still, then?" he asked, and in his voice was blent all the exultation, and the wonder, and the piercing torment of love itself.

Sara felt herself slipping, knew that she was losing her hold of herself. Soon she would be a-wash in a sea of love, helpless to resist as a bit of driftwood, and then the waters would close over her head and she would be drawn down into the depths of shame which yielding to her love for Garth involved.

She must go--leave him while she had the power. Summoning up her strength, she faced him.

"I do," she answered steadily. "But I pray God every night of my life that I may soon cease to care."

And with those few words, limitless in their scorn--for him, and for herself because she still loved him--she turned to go.

But their contempt seemed to pass him by. His eyes burned.

"So Elisabeth has played her stake--and lost!" he muttered to himself. "Ah! Par-don!" he drew aside as she almost brushed past him in her sudden haste to escape--to get away--and stood, with bared head, his eyes fixed on her receding figure.

Soon a bend in the path through the fields hid her from his sight. But, long after she had disappeared, he remained leaning, motionless, against the gateway through which she had passed, his face immobile, twisted and drawn so that it resembled some sculptured mask of Pain, his eyes staring straight in front of him, blank and unseeing.

"Hullo, Trent!"

Miles Herrick, returning from the town to the hospital and taking, like every one else, the short cut across the fields, waved a friendly arm as he caught sight of Garth's figure silhouetted against the sky-line.

Then he drew nearer, and the set, still face of the other filled him with a sudden sense of dismay. There was a new look in it, a kind of dogged hopelessness. It entirely lacked that suggestion of austere sweetness which had made it so difficult to reconcile his smirched reputation with the man himself.

"What is it, Garth?" Instinctively Miles slipped into the more familiar appellation.

Trent looked at him blankly. It seemed as though he had not heard the question, or, at any rate, had not taken in its meaning.

"What did you say?" he muttered, his brows contracting painfully.

Miles slung the various packages with which he was burdened on to the ground, and leaned up leisurely against the gatepost. It was characteristic of him that, although the day was never long enough for the work he crowded into it, he could always find time to give a helping hand to a pal with his back against the wall.

"Out with it, man!" he said. "What's up?"

Slowly recognition came back in the other's eyes.

"What I might have anticipated," he answered, at last, in a curious flat voice, devoid of expression. "I've sunk a degree or two lower in Sara's estimation since the war broke out."

Miles regarded him quietly for a moment, a queer, half-humorous glint in his eyes.

"I suppose she doesn't know you've half-beggared yourself, helping on the financial side?"

"A man could hardly do less, could he?" he returned awkwardly. "But if she did know--which she doesn't--it would make no earthly difference."

"Then--it's because you're not soldiering?"

"Exactly. I've not volunteered."

"Well"--composedly--"why don't you?"

Trent laughed shortly.

"That's my affair."

"With your physique you could wangle the age limit," pursued Miles imperturbably.

"I should have to 'wangle' a good deal more than that,"--harshly. "Have you forgotten that I was chucked from the Army?"

"There's such a thing as enlisting under another name."

"There is--and then of running up against one of the old crowd and being recognized! It isn't so easy to lose your identity. I've had my lesson on that."

Miles looked away quickly. The hard, implacable stare of the other man's eyes, with the blazing defiance, hurt him. It spoke too poignantly of a bitterness that had eaten into the heart. But he had put his hand to the plough, and he refused to turn back.

"Wouldn't it"--he spoke with a sudden gentleness, the gentleness of the surgeon handling a torn limb--"wouldn't it help to straighten things out with Sara?"

"If it did, it would only make matters worse. No. Take it from me, Herrick, that soldiering is the one thing of all others I can't do."

He turned away as though to signify that the discussion was at an end.

"I don't see it," persisted Miles. "On the contrary, it's the one thing that might make her believe in you. In spite of that Indian Frontier business."

Garth swung suddenly round, a dull, dangerous gleam in his eyes. But Miles bore the savage glance serenely. He had applied the spur with intention. The other was suffering--suffering intolerably--in a dumb silence that shut him in alone with his agony. That silence must be broken, no matter what the means.

"You'd wipe out the stigma of cowardice, if you volunteered," he went on deliberately.

Garth laughed derisively.

"Cut it out, Herrick," he flung back. "I'm not a damned story-book hero, out for whitewash and the V.C."

But Miles continued undeterred.

"And you'd convince Sara," he finished quietly.

A stifled exclamation broke from Garth.

"To what end?" he burst out violently. "Can't you realize that's just the one thing in the world forbidden me? Sara is--oh, well, it's impossible to say what she is, but I suppose most good women are half angel. And if I gave her the smallest chance, she'd begin to believe in me again--to ask questions I cannot answer. . . .

What's the use? I can't get away from the court-martial and all that followed. I can't clear myself. And I could never offer Sara anything more than a name that has been disgraced--a miserable half-life with a man who can't hold up his head amongst his fellows! Yes"--answering the unspoken question in Herrick's eyes--"I know what you're thinking--that I was willing to marry her once. But I believed, then, that--Garth Trent had cut himself free from the past. Now I know"--more quietly--"that there is no such thing as getting away from the mistakes one has made. . . . I'm tied hand and foot--every way! And it's better Sara should continue to think the worst of me. Then, in the future, she may find some sort of happiness--with Durward, perhaps." His lips greyed a little, but he went on. "The worse she thinks me, the easier it will be for her to cut me out of her life."

"Then do you mean"--Miles spoke very slowly--"that you are--deliberately--holding back from soldiering?"

"Quite deliberately!" It was like the snap of a tormented animal, baited beyond bearing. "If I could go with a clean name, as other men can----Good God, man! Do you think I haven't thought it out--knocked my head against every stone wall in the whole damned business?"

Miles was silent. There was so much of truth in all Garth said, so much of warped vision, biased by the man's profound bitterness of soul, that he could find no answer.

After a moment Garth spoke again, jerkily, as though under pressure.

"There's my promise to Elisabeth, as well. That binds me if I were recognized and taxed with my identity. I should have to hold my peace--and stick it all over again! . . . There's a limit to a man's endurance."

Then, after a pause: "If I could go--and be sure of not returning"--grimly--"I'd go to-morrow--the Foreign Legion, anyway. But sometimes a man hasn't even the right to get himself neatly killed out of the way."

"What are you driving at now?"

"I should think it's plain enough! Don't you see what it would mean to Sara if--that--happened? She'd never believe--afterwards--that I'm as black as I'm painted, and I should saddle her with an intolerable burden of self-reproach. No, the Army is a closed door for me. . . . Damn it, Herrick!" with the sudden nervous violence of a man goaded past endurance. "Can't you understand? I ought never to have come into her life at all. I've only messed things up for her--damnably. The least I can do is to clear out of it so that she'll never regret my going. . . . I've gone under, and a man who's gone under had better stay there."

Both men were silent--Trent with the bitter, brooding silence of a man who has battered uselessly against the bars that hem him in, and who at last recognizes that they can never be forced asunder, Herrick trying to focus his vision to that of the man beside him.

"No"--Garth spoke with a finality there was no disputing--"I've been buried three-and-twenty years, and my resurrection hasn't been exactly a success. There's no place in the world for me unless some one else pays the price. It's better for every one concerned that I should--stay buried."

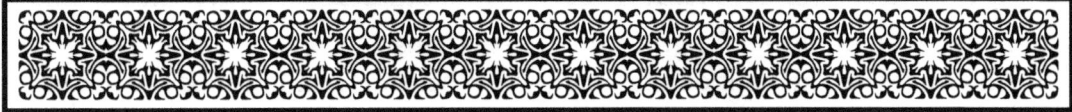

CHAPTER XXXIII
OVER THE MOUNTAINS

H e didn't do it!"

Suddenly, Sara found herself saying the words aloud in the darkness and solitude of the night.

Since her meeting with Garth, on her way to the hospital, every hour had been an hour of conflict. That brief, strained interview had shaken her to the depths of her being, and, unable to sleep when night came, she had lain, staring wide-eyed into the dark, struggling against its influence.

Little enough had been said. It had been the silences, the dumb, passion-filled silences, vibrant with all that must not be spoken, which had tried her endurance to the utmost, and she had fled, at last, incontinently, because she had felt her resolution weakening each moment she and Garth remained together--because, with him beside her, the love against which she had been fighting for twelve long months had wakened into fierce life again, beating down her puny efforts to withstand it.

The mere sound of his voice, the lightest touch of his hand, had power to thrill her from head to foot, to rock those barriers which his own act had forced her to build up between them.

The recollection of that one perfect moment, when the serene austerity of his face had given the lie to that of which he was accused, lingered with her, a faint elusive thread of hope which would not leave her, urging, suggesting, combating the hard facts to which he himself had given ruthless confirmation.

Almost without her cognizance, Sara's characteristic, vehement belief in whomsoever she loved--stunned at the first moment of Elisabeth's revelation--had been gradually creeping back to feeble, halting life, weakened at times by the mass of evidence arrayed against it, yet still alive--growing and strengthening secretly within her as an unborn babe grows and strengthens.

And since that moment on the moor, when her eyes had searched Garth's face--his face with the mask off--the dormant belief within her had sprung into conscious knowledge.

Throughout the long hours of the night she had fought against it, deeming it but the passionate outcome of her love for the man himself. She **wanted** to believe him innocent; it was only her love for him which had raised this phantom doubt of the charges brought against him; the wish had been father to the thought. So she told herself, struggling conscientiously against that to which she longed to yield.

And then, making a mockery of the hateful thing of which he had been accused, her individual knowledge of Garth himself rose up and confronted her accusingly.

Nothing that she had ever known of him had pointed to any lack of courage. It had been on no sudden, splendid impulse of a moment that he had plunged into the sea and fought that treacherous, racing tide off Devil's Hood Island. Quite composedly, deliberately, he had calculated the risks--and taken them!

Once more, she recalled the vision of his face as she had seen it yesterday, in that instant before he had perceived her nearness to him--strong and steadfast, imprinted with a disciplined nobility--and the repudiation of his dishonour leapt spontaneously from her lips.

"He didn't do it!"

She had spoken involuntarily, the thought rushing into words before she was aware, and the sound of her own voice in the darkness startled her. It seemed almost like a voice from some Otherwhere, authoritatively assuring her of all she had ached to believe.

She lay back on her pillows, smiling a little at the illusion. But the sense of peace, of blessed assuredness, remained with her. She had struggled through the darkness of those bitter months of unbelief, and now she had come out into the light on the other side. She felt dreamily contented and at rest, and presently she fell asleep, trustfully, as a little child may sleep, the smile still on her lips.

With morning came reaction--blank, sordid reaction, depressing her unutterably.

Amid the score of trifling details incidental to the day's arrangements, with the usual uninspiring conversation prevalent at the breakfast-table going on around her, the mood of the previous night, informed, as it had been, with that triumphant sense of exaltation, slipped from her like a garment.

Supposing she were to tell them--to tell Selwyn and Molly--that, without any further evidence, she was convinced of Garth's innocence? Why, they would think she had gone mad! Regretfully, with infinite pain it might be, but still none the less conclusively, they had accepted the fact of his guilt. And indeed, what else could be expected of them, seeing that he had himself acknowledged it?

And yet--that inner feeling of belief which had stirred into new life refused to be repressed.

Mechanically she went about the small daily duties which made up life at Sunnyside--interviewed Jane Crab, read the newspapers to Mrs. Selwyn, accomplished the necessary shopping in the town, each and all with a mind that was only superficially concerned with the matter in hand, while, behind this screen of commonplace routine, she felt as though her soul were struggling impotently to release itself from the bonds which had bound it in a tyranny of anguish for twelve long months.

In the afternoon, she paid a visit to the Convalescent Hospital. She made a practice of going there at least once a day and giving what assistance she could. Frequently she relieved Miles of part of his secretarial work, or checked through with him the invoices of goods received. There were always plenty of odd jobs to be done, and, after her strenuous work in France, she found it utterly impossible to settle down to the life of masterly inactivity which Selwyn had prescribed for her.

Audrey greeted her with a little flurry of excitement.

"Do you know that there was a Zepp over Oldhampton last night?" she asked, as they went upstairs together. "Did you hear it?"

Sara shook her head. The memory of the previous night surged over her like the memory of a vivid dream--the absolute assurance it had brought her of Garth's innocence, an assurance which had grown vague and doubtful with the daylight, just as the happenings of a dream grow blurred and indistinct.

"No, I didn't hear anything," she replied absently. "Did they do much damage? I suppose they were after the munitions factory?"

"Yes. They dropped one bomb, that's all. It fell in a field, luckily. But goodness knows how they got over without any one's spotting them! Everybody's asking where our search-lights were. As for our anti-aircraft guns, they've never had the opportunity yet to do anything more than try our nerves by practicing! And last night a golden opportunity came and went unobserved."

"The milkman was babbling to Jane about Zeppelins this morning, but I thought it was probably only the result of overnight potations at 'The Jolly Sailorman.'"

"No, it was the real thing--'made in Germany,'" smiled Audrey. "I begin to feel as if we were quite the hub of the universe, now that the Zepps have acknowledged our existence."

They paused outside the door of the room allotted to her husband's activities.

"Miles will be glad to see you to-day," she pursued. "He's bemoaning a new manifestation of war-fever among the feminine population of Monkshaven. Go in to him, will you? I must run off--I've got a million things to see to. You're not looking very fit to-day"--suddenly observing the other's white face and shadowed eyes. "Are you feeling up to work?"

Sara nodded indifferently.

"Quite," she said. "I shouldn't have come otherwise."

Miles welcomed her joyfully.

"Bless you, my dear!" he exclaimed. "You're the very woman I wanted to see. I'm snowed under with fool letters from females anxious to entertain 'our poor, brave, wounded officers.' Head 'em off, will you?" He thrust a bundle of letters into her hands. Then, as she moved toward the windows, and the cold, searching light of the wintry sunshine fell full on her face, his voice altered. "What is it? What has happened, Sara?" he asked quickly.

She looked at him dumbly. Her lips moved, but no sound came. The sudden question, accompanied by the swift, penetrating glance of Miles's brown eyes, had taken her off her guard.

He limped across to her.

"Not a stroke of work for you to-day," he said decisively, taking the bundle of letters out of her hands. "Now tell me what's wrong?"

She looked away from him, a slow, shamed red creeping into her face. At last--

"I've seen Garth," she said very low.

Herrick nodded. He knew what that meeting had meant to one of these two friends of his. Now he was to see the reverse of the medal. He waited, his silence sympathetic and far more helpful than any eager, probing question, however well-intentioned.

"Miles," she burst out suddenly, "I'm--I'm wretched!"

"How's that?" He did not make the mistake of attributing her outburst to a transient mood of depression. Something deeper lay behind it.

"Since I saw Garth yesterday I've been asking myself whether--whether I've been doing him a ghastly injustice"--she moistened her dry lips--"whether he was really guilty of--running away."

"Ah!" Miles stuffed his hands in his pockets and limped the length of the room and back. In that moment, he realized something of the maddening, galling restraint of the bondage under which Garth Trent had lived for years--the bondage of silence, and, within his pickets, his hands were clenched when he halted again at Sara's side.

"Why?" he shot at her.

She hesitated. Then she caught her breath a little hysterically.

"Why--because--because I just can't believe it! . . . I've seen a lot since I went away. I've seen brave men--and I've seen men . . . who were afraid." She turned her head aside. "They--the ones who were afraid--didn't look . . . as Garth looks."

Herrick made no comment. He put a question.

"What are you going to do?"

"I don't know. I expect you think I'm a fool? I've nothing to go on--on the contrary, I've Garth's own admission that--that he *was* cashiered. And yet----Oh! Miles, if he were only doing anything--now--it would be easier to believe in him! But--he holds absolutely aloof. It's as though he *were* afraid--still."

"Have you ever thought"--Herrick spoke slowly, without looking at her--"what this year of war must have meant to a man who has been a soldier--and is one no longer?" His eyes came back to her face meditatively.

"How--what do you mean?" she whispered.

"You've only got to look at the man to know what I mean. I think--since the war broke out--that Trent has been through the bitterness of death."

"But--but he could have enlisted--got in somehow--under another name, had he *wanted* to fight. Or he might have gone out and driven an ambulance car--as Lester Kent did."

Sara was putting to Herrick the very arguments which had arisen in her own mind to confound the intuitive belief of which she had been conscious since that moment of inward revelation on Crabtree Moor--putting them forward in all their repulsive ugliness of fact, in the desperate hope that Herrick might find some way to refute them.

"Some men might have done, perhaps," answered Miles quietly. "But not a man of Trent's temperament. Some trees bend in a storm--and when the worst of it is past, they spring erect again. Some *can't*; they break."

The words recalled to Sara's mind with sudden vividness the last letter Patrick Lovell had ever written her--the one which he had left in the Chippendale bureau for her to receive after his death. He had applied almost those identical words to the Malincourt temperament, of which he had recognized the share she had inherited. And she realized that her guardian and Miles Herrick had been equally discerning. Though differing in its effect upon each of them, consequent upon individual idiosyncrasy, the fact remained that she and Garth were both "breaking" beneath the strain which destiny had imposed on them.

With the memory of Patrick's letter came an inexpressible longing for the man himself--for the kindly, helping hand which he would have stretched out to her in this crisis of her life. She felt sure that, had he been beside her now, his shrewd counsel would have cleared away the mists of doubt and indecision which had closed about her.

But since he was no longer there to be appealed to, she had turned instinctively to Herrick, and, somehow, he had failed her. He had not given her a definite expression of his own belief. She had been humanly craving to hear that he, too, believed in Garth, notwithstanding the evidence against him--that he had some explanation to offer of that ghastly tragedy of the court-martial episode. And instead, he had only hazarded some tolerant suggestions--sympathetic to Garth, it is true, but not carrying with them the vital, unqualified assurance she had longed to hear.

In spite of this, she knew that Herrick's friendship with Garth had remained unbroken by the knowledge of the Indian Frontier story. The personal relations of the two men were unchanged, and she felt as though Miles were withholding something from her, observing a reticence for which she could find no explanation. He had been very kind and understanding--it would not have been Miles had he been otherwise--but he had not helped her much. In some curious way she felt as though he had thrown the whole onus of coming to a decision, unaided by advice, upon her shoulders.

She returned to Sunnyside oppressed with a homesick longing for Patrick. The two years which had elapsed since his death had blunted the edge of her sorrow--as time inevitably must--but she still missed the shrewd, kindly, worldly-wise old man unspeakably, and just now, thrown back upon herself in some indefinable way by Miles's attitude, her whole heart cried out for that other who was gone.

She wondered if he knew how much she needed him. She almost believed that he must know--wherever he might be now, she felt that Patrick would never have forgotten the child of the woman whom, in this world, he had loved so long and faithfully.

With an instinctive craving for some tangible memory of him, she unlocked the leather case which held her mother's miniature, together with the last letter which Patrick had ever written; and, unfolding the letter, began to read it once again.

Somehow, there seemed comfort in the very wording of it, in every little characteristic phrase that had been Patrick's, in the familiar appellation, "Little old pal," which he had kept for her alone.

All at once her fingers gripped the letter more tightly, her attentions riveted by a certain passage towards the end.

". . . And when love comes to you, never forget that it is the biggest thing in the world, the one altogether good and perfect gift. Don't let any twopenny-halfpenny considerations of worldly advantage influence you, or the tittle-tattle of other folks, and even if it seems that something unsurmountable lies between you and the fulfillment of love, go over it, or round it, or through it! If it's real love, your faith must be big enough to remove the mountains in the way--or to go over them."

Had Patrick foreseen the exact circumstances in which his "little old pal" would one day find herself, he could not have written anything more strangely applicable.

Sara sat still, every nerve of her taut and strung. She felt as though she had laid bare the whole of her trouble, revealed her inmost soul in all its anguished perplexity, to those shrewd blue eyes which had been wont to see so clearly through externals, piercing infallibly to the very heart of things.

Patrick had always possessed that supreme gift of being able to separate the grain from the chaff--to distinguish unerringly between essentials and non-essentials, and now, in the quiet, wise counsel of an old letter, Sara found an answer to all the questionings that had made so bitter a thing of life.

It was almost as if some one had torn down a curtain from before her eyes, rent asunder a veil which had been distorting and obscuring the values of things.

Mountains! There were mountains indeed betwixt her and Garth--and there was no way round them or through them! But now--now she would go over them--go straight ahead, unregarding of the mountains between, to where Garth and love awaited her.

No man is all angel--or all devil. Supposing Garth *had* been guilty of cowardice, had had his one moment of weakness? She no longer cared! He was hers, her lover, alike in his weakness and in his strength. She had known men in France shrink in terror at the evil droning of a shell, and then die selflessly that others might live.

"Your faith must be big enough to remove the mountains in the way--or to go over them," Patrick had written.

And Sara, hiding her face in her hands, thanked God that now, at last, her faith was big enough, and that love--"the one altogether good and perfect gift"--was still hers if she would only go over the mountains.

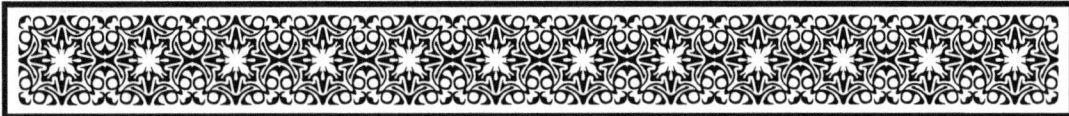

CHAPTER XXXIV
THE TRIUMPH OF LOVE
"GARTH TRENT, COWARD."

The words, in staring white capital letters, had been chalked up by some one on the big wooden double-doors that shut the world out from Far End. Sara stood quite still, gazing at them fixedly, and a tense white-heat of anger flared up within her. Who had dared to put such an insult upon the man she loved?

"*Coward*!" No one had ever actually applied that term to Garth in her hearing. They had skirted delicately round it, or wrapped up its meaning in some less harsh-sounding tangle of phrases, and although she had bitterly used the word herself, now that the opprobrious expression publicly confronted her, writ large by some unfriendly hand, she was swept by a sheer fury of indignant denial. It roused in her the immediate instinct to defend, to range herself unmistakably on Garth's side against a world of traducers.

With a faint smile of self-mockery, she realized that had this flagrant insult been leveled at him in the beginning, had her first knowledge of the black shadow which hung over him been thus brutally flung at her, instead of diffidently, reluctantly broken to her by Elisabeth, she would probably, with the instinctive partisanship of woman for her mate, have utterly refused to credit it--against all reason and all proof.

She wondered who could have done this ting, nailed this insult to Garth's very door. The illiterate characters stamped it as the work of some one in the lower walks of life, and, with a frown of annoyance, Sara promptly--and quite correctly--ascribed it to Black Brady.

"I never forgits to pay back," he had told her once, belligerently. Probably this was his notion of getting even with the man who had prosecuted him for poaching. But had Brady realized that, in retaliating upon Trent, he would be giving pain to his beloved Sara, whom he had grown to regard with a humble, dog-like devotion, he would certainly have refrained from recording his vengeance upon Garth's gateway.

Surmising that Garth could not have seen the offending legend--or it would scarcely have been left for all who can to read--Sara whipped out her handkerchief and set to work to rub it off. He should not see it if she could help it!

But Black Brady had done his work very thoroughly, and she was still diligently scrubbing at it with an inadequate piece of cambric when she heard steps behind her, and wheeling round, found herself confronted by Garth himself.

His eyes rested indifferently and without surprise upon the chalked-up words, then turned to Sara's face inquiringly.

"Why are you doing that?" he asked. "Is--cleaning gates the latest form of war-work?"

Sara, her face scarlet, answered reluctantly.

"I didn't want you to see it."

A curious expression flashed into his eyes.

"I saw it--two hours ago."

"And you left it there?"--with amazement.

"Why not? It's true, isn't it?"

And in that moment the long struggle in Sara's heart ended, and she answered out of the fullness of the faith that was in her.

"No! It is **not** true! I've been a fool to believe it for an instant. But I'm one no longer. I don't believe it." She paused, then, very deliberately and steadily, she put her question.

"Garth--tell me, were you ever guilty of cowardice?"

"The court-martial thought so."

Sara's foot tapped impatiently on the ground.

"Please answer my question," she said quickly.

But he remained unmoved.

"Elisabeth Durward has surely supplied you with all the information on that subject which you require," he said in expressionless tones, and Sara was conscious anew of the maddening feeling of impotence with which a contest of wills between herself and Garth never failed to imbue her.

"Garth"--there was appeal in her voice, yet it was still very steady and determined--"I want to know what *you* say about it. What Elisabeth--or any one else--may say, doesn't matter any longer."

Something in the quiet depth of emotion in her voice momentarily broke through his guard. He made an involuntary movement towards her, then checked himself, and, with an effort, resumed his former detached manner.

"More important than anything either I, or Elisabeth, can say, is the verdict of the court," he answered.

The deadly calm of his voice ripped away her last remnant of composure.

"The verdict of the court!" she burst out. "***Damn*** the verdict of the court!"

"I have done--many a time!"--bitterly.

"Garth," she came a step nearer to him and her sombre eyes blazed into his. "I *will* have an answer! For God's sake, don't fence with me any longer! . . . There have been misunderstandings enough, reticences enough, between us. For this once, let us be honest with each other. I pretended I didn't care--I pretended I could go on living, believing you to be what--what they have called you. And I can't! . . . I can't go on. . . . I can't bear it any longer. You must answer me! ***Were you guilty?***"

He was white to the lips by the time she had finished, and his eyes held a look of dumb torture. Twice he essayed to answer her, but no sound came.

At last he turned away, as though the passionate question in her face--the eager, hungry longing to hear her faith confirmed--were more than he could bear.

"I cannot deny it." The words came hoarsely, almost whispered.

Her eyes never left his face.

"I didn't ask you to deny it," she persisted doggedly. "I asked you--were you guilty?"

Again there fell as heavy silence. Then, reluctantly, as if the admission were dragged from him, he spoke.

"I'm afraid I can give you no other answer to that question."

A light like the tender, tremulous shining of dawn broke across Sara's face.

"Then you ***weren't*** guilty!" she exclaimed, and there was a deep, surpassing joy in her shaken tones. "I knew it! I was sure of it. Oh! Garth, Garth, what a fool I've been! And oh! My dear, why did you do it? Why did you let me go on thinking you--what it almost killed me to think?"

He stared down at her with wondering, uncertain eyes.

"But I've just told you that I can't deny it!"

She smiled at him--a smile of absolute content, with a gleam of humour at the back of it.

"I didn't ask you to deny it. I asked you to own to it; I tried to make you--every way. And you can't!"

"But--"

She laid her hand across his mouth--laughing the tender, triumphant laughter of a woman who has won, and knows that she has.

"You needn't blacken yourself any longer on my account, Garth. I shall never again believe anything that you may say against--the man I love."

She stood leaning a little towards him, surrender in every line of her slender body, and her face was like a white flame--transfigured, radiant with some secret, mystic glory of love's imparting.

With an inarticulate cry he opened wide his arms and she went to him--swiftly, unerringly, like a homing bird--and, as he folded her close against his breast and laid his lips to hers, all the hunger and the longing of the empty past was in his kiss. For the moment, pain and bitterness and regret were swept away in that ecstasy of reunion.

Presently, with a little sigh of spent rapture, she leaned away from him.

"To think we've wasted a whole year," she said regretfully. "Garth, I wish I had trusted you better!" There was a sweet humility of repentance in her tones.

"I don't see why you should trust me now," he rejoined quietly. "The facts remain as before."

"Only that the verdict of the court-martial was wrong," she said swiftly. "There was some horrible mistake. I am sure of it--I know it! Garth!"--after a moment's pause--"are you going to tell me everything? I have the right to know--haven't I?--now that I'm going to be your wife."

She felt the clasp of his arms relax, and, looking up quickly, she saw his face suddenly revert to its old lines of weariness. Slowly, reluctantly, he drew away from her.

"Garth!" There was a shrilling note of apprehension in her voice. "Garth! What is it? Why do you look like that?"

It was a full minute before he answered. When he did, he spoke heavily, as one who knows that his next words will dash all the joy out of life.

"Because," he said quietly, "I can no more tell you anything now than I could before. I can't clear myself, Sara!"

Her eyes were fixed on his.

"Do you mean--you will *never* be able to?" she asked incredulously.

"Yes, I mean that."

"Answer me one more question, Garth. Is it that you *cannot*--or *will not* clear yourself?"

"I *must* not," he replied steadily. "I am not the only one concerned in the matter. There is some one to whom I owe it to be silent. Honour forbids that I should even try to clear myself. Now you know all--all that I can ever tell you."

"Who is it?" The question leaped from her, and Garth's answer came with an irrevocability of refusal there was no combating.

"That I cannot tell you--or any one."

Sara's mouth twitched. Her face was very white, but her eyes were shining.

"And you have borne this--all these years?" she said. "You have known that you could clear yourself and have refrained?"

"There was no choice," he answered quietly. "I took on a certain liability--years ago, and because it has turned out to be a much heavier liability than I anticipated gives me no excuse for repudiating it now."

For a moment Sara hid her face in her hands. When she uncovered it again there was something almost akin to awe in her eyes.

"Will you ever forgive me, Garth, for doubting you?" she whispered.

"Forgive you?" He smiled. "What else could you have done, sweetheart? I don't know, even now, why you believe in me," he added wonderingly.

"Just because--" she began, and fell silent, realizing that her belief had no reason, but was founded on the intuitive knowledge of a love that has suffered and won out on the other side.

When next she spoke it was with the simple, frank directness characteristic of her.

"Thank God that I can prove that I do trust you--absolutely. When will you marry me, Garth?"

"When will I marry you?" He repeated the words slowly, as though they conveyed no meaning to him.

"Yes. I want every one to know, to see that I believe in you. I want to stand at your side--go shares. Do you remember, once, how we settled that married life meant going shares in everything--good and bad?" She smiled a little at the remembrance drawn from the small store of memories that was all her few days of unclouded love had given her. "I want--my share, Garth."

For a moment he was silent. Then he spoke, and the quiet finality of his tones struck her like a blow.

"We can never marry, Sara."

"Never--marry!" she repeated dazedly. Quick fear seized her, and she rushed on impetuously: "Then you haven't forgiven me, after all--you don't believe that I trust you! Oh! How can I make you *know* that I do? Garth--"

"Oh, my dear," he interrupted swiftly. "Don't misunderstand me. I know that you believe in me now--and I thank God for it! And as for forgiveness, as I told you, I have nothing to forgive. You'd have had need of the faith that removes mountains"--Sara started at the repetition of Patrick's very words--"to have believed in me under the circumstances." He paused a moment, and when he spoke again there was something triumphant in his tones--a serene gladness and contentment. "You and I, beloved, are right with each other--now and always. Nothing can ever again come between us to divide us as we have been divided this last year. But, none the less," and his voice took on a steadfast note of resolve, "I cannot marry you. I thought I could--I thought the past had sunk into oblivion, and that I might take the gift of love you offered me. . . . But I was wrong."

"No! No! You were not wrong!" She was clinging to him in a sudden terror that even now their happiness was slipping from them. "The past has nothing to say to you and me. It can't come between us. . . . You have only to take me, Garth"-- tremulously. "Let me *show* that my love is stronger than ill repute. Let me come to you and stand by you as your wife. The past can't hurt us, then!"

He shook his head.

"The past never loses its power to hurt," he answered. "I've learned that. As far as the world you belong to is concerned, I'm finished, and I won't drag the woman I love through the same hell I've been through. That's what it would mean, you know. You would be singled out, pointed at, as the wife of a man who was chucked out of the Service. There would be no place in the world for you. You would be ostracized--because you were my wife."

"I shouldn't care," she urged. "Surely I can bear--what you have borne? . . . I shouldn't mind--anything--so long as we were together."

He drew her close to him, his lips against her hair.

"Beloved!" he said, a great wonder in his voice. "Oh! Little **brave** thing! What have I ever done that you should love me like that?"

Sara winked away a tear, and a rather tremulous smile hovered round her mouth.

"I don't know, I'm sure," she acknowledged a little shakily. "But I do. Garth, you *will* marry me?"

He lifted his bent head, his eyes gazing straight ahead of him, as though envisioning the lonely future and defying it.

"No," he said resolutely. "No. God helping me, I will never marry you, Sara. I have--no right to marry. It could only bring you misery. Dear, I must shield you, even from yourself--from your own big, generous impulses which would let you join your life to mine. . . . Love is denied to us--denied through my own act of long ago. But if you'll give me friendship. . . ." She could sense the sudden passionate entreaty behind the words. "Sara! Friendship is worth while--such friendship as ours would be! Are you brave enough, strong enough, to give me that--since I may not ask for more?"

There was a long silence, while Sara lay very still against his breast, her face hidden.

In that silence, her spirit met and faced the ultimate issue--for there was that in Garth's voice which told her that his decision not to marry her was immutable. Could she--oh God!--could she give him what he asked? Give only part to the man to whom she longed to give all that a woman has to give? It would be far easier to go away--to put him out of her life for ever.

And yet--he asked this of her! He needed something that she could still give--

the comradeship which was all that they two might ever know of love. . . .

When at last she raised her face to his, it was ashen, but her small chin was out-thrust, her eyes were like stars, and the grip of her slim hands on his shoulders was as iron.

"I'm strong enough to give you anything that you want," she said quietly.

She had made the supreme sacrifice; she was ready to be his friend.

A sad and wistful gravity hung about their parting. Their lips met and clung together, but it was in a kiss of renunciation, not of passion.

He held her in his arms a moment longer.

"Never forget I'm loving you--always," he said steadily. "Call me your friend-- but remember, in my heart I shall always be your lover."

Her eyes met his, unflinching, infinitely faithful.

"And I--I, too, shall be loving you," she answered, simply. "Always, Garth-- always."

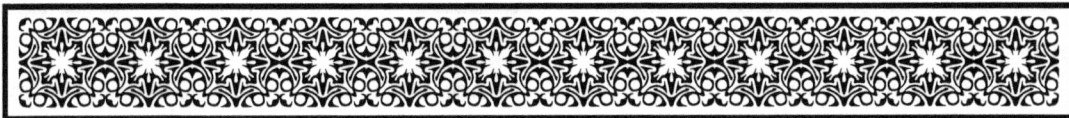

CHAPTER XXXV
OUT OF THE NIGHT

Tim was home on sick leave, and, after two perfect weeks of reunion, Elisabeth had written to ask if he might come down to Sunnyside, suggesting that the sea-breezes might advance his convalescence.

"I wonder Mrs. Durward cares to spare him," commented Selwyn in some surprise. "It seems out of keeping with her general attitude. However, we shall be delighted to have him here. Write and say so, will you, Sara?"

Sara acquiesced briefly, flushing a little. She thought she could read the motive at the back of Elisabeth's proposal--the spirit which, putting up a gallant fight even in the very face of defeat, could make yet a final effort to secure success by throwing Tim and the woman he loved together in the dangerously seductive intimacy of the same household.

But Sara had no fear that Tim would avail himself of the opportunity thus provided in the way Elisabeth doubtless hoped he might. That matter had been finally settled between herself and him before he went to France, and she knew that he would never again ask her to be his wife. So she wrote to him serenely, telling him to come down to Monkshaven as soon as he liked; and a few days later found him installed at Sunnyside, nominally under Dr. Selwyn's care.

He was the same unaffected, spontaneous Tim as of yore, and hugely embarrassed by any reference to his winning of the Military Cross, firmly refusing to discuss the manner of it, even with Sara.

"I just got on with my job--like dozens of other fellows," was all he would say.

It was from a brother officer that Sara learned, later, than Tim had "got on with his job" under a hellish enemy fire, in spite of being twice wounded; and had thus saved the immediate situation in his vicinity--and, incidentally, the lives of many of his comrades.

He seemed to Sara to have become at once both older and younger than in former days. He had all the hilarious good spirits evinced by nine out of ten of the boys who came home on leave--the cheery capacity to laugh at the hardships and dangers of the front, to poke good-natured fun at "old Fritz" and to make a jest of the German shells and the Flanders mud, treating the whole great adventure of war as though it were the finest game invented.

Yet back of the mirth and laughter in the blue eyes lurked something new and strange and grave--inexpressibly touching--that indefinable something which one senses shrinkingly in the young eyes of the boys who have come back.

It hurt Sara somehow--that look of which she caught glimpses now and then, in quiet moments, and she set herself to drive it away, or, at least, to keep it at bay as much as possible, by filling every available moment with occupation or amusement.

"I don't want him to think about what it was like--out there," she told Molly. "His eyes make my heart ache, sometimes. They're too young to have seen--such things. Suggest something we can play at to-day!"

So they threw themselves, heart and soul, into the task of entertaining Tim, and, since he was very willing to be entertained, the weeks at Sunnyside slipped by in a little whirl of gaiety, winding up with a badminton tournament, at which Tim--whose right arm had not yet quite recovered from the effects of the German bullet it had stopped--played a left-handed game, and triumphantly maneuvered himself and his partner into the semi-finals.

Probably--leniently handicapped, as they were, in the circumstances--they would have won the tournament, but that, unluckily, in leaping to reach a shuttle soaring high above his head, Tim somehow missed his footing and came down heavily, with his leg twisted underneath him.

"Broken ankle," announced Selwyn briefly, when he had made his examination.

Tim opened his eyes--he had lost consciousness, momentarily, from the pain.

"Damn!" he observed succinctly. "That'll make it the very devil of a time before I can get back to France!" Then, to Sara, who could be heard murmuring something about writing to Elisabeth: "Not much, old thing, you don't! She'd fuss herself, no end. Just write--and say--it's a sprain." And he promptly fainted again.

They got him back to Sunnyside while he was still unconscious, and when he returned to an intelligent understanding of material matters, he found himself in bed, with a hump-like excrescence in front of him keeping the weight of the bed-clothes from the injured limb.

"Did I faint?" he asked morosely.

"Yes. Lucky you did, too," responded Sara cheerfully. "Doctor Dick rigged your ankle up all nice and comfy without your being any the wiser."

"Fainted--like a girl--over a broken ankle, my hat!"--with immense scorn.

Sara was hard put to it not to laugh outright at his face of disgust.

"You might remember that you're not strong yet," she suggested soothingly.

They talked for a little, and presently Tim, whose eyelids had been blinking somnolently for some time, gave vent to an unmistakable yawn.

"I'm--I'm confoundedly sleepy," he murmured apologetically.

"Then go to sleep," came promptly from Sara. "It's quite the best thing you can do. I'll run off and write a judicious letter to Elisabeth--about your sprain"--smiling.

With a glance round to see that he had candle, matches, and a hand-bell within reach, she turned out the lamp and slipped quietly away. Tim was asleep almost before she had quitted the room.

It was several hours later when Sara sat up in bed, broad awake, in response to the vigorous shaking that some one was administering to her.

She opened her eyes to the yellow glare of a candle. Behind the glare material-ized a vision of Jane Crab, attired in a red flannel dressing-gown, and with her hair tightly strained into four skimpy plaits which stuck out horizontally from her head like the surviving rays of a badly damaged halo.

"Miss Sara! Miss Sara!" She apostrophized the rudely awakened sleeper in a sibilant whisper, as though afraid of being overheard. "Get up, quick! They 'Uns is 'ere!"

"*Who* is here?" exclaimed Sara, somewhat startled.

"The Zepps, miss--the Zepps! The guns are firing off every minute or two. There!"--as the blurred thunder of anti-aircraft guns boomed in the distance. "There they go again!"

Sara leaped out of bed in an instant, hastily pulling on a fascinating silk kimono and thrusting her bare feet into a pair of scarlet Turkish slippers.

"One may as well die tidy," she reflected philosophically. Then, turning to Jane--

"Where's the doctor?" she demanded.

"Trying to get the mistress downstairs. She's that scared, she won't budge from her bed."

Sara giggled--Jane's face was very expressive.

"Well, I'm going into Mr. Durward's room," she announced. "We shall see better there."

Jane's little beady eyes glittered.

"Aye, I'd like to see them at their devil's work," she allowed fondly, with a threatening "Just-let-me-catch-them-at-it!" intonation in her voice.

Sara laughed, and they both repaired to Tim's room, encountering Molly on the way and sweeping her along in their train. They found Tim volubly cursing his inability to get up and "watch the fun."

"Look out and tell me if you can see the blighters," he commanded.

As Sara threw open the window, a dull, thudding sound came up to them from the direction of Oldhampton. There was a sullen menace in the distance-dulled reverberation.

Molly gurgled with the nervous excitement of a first experience under fire.

"That's a bomb!" she whispered breathlessly.

She, and Sara, and Jane Crab wedged themselves together in the open window and leaned far out, peering into the moonless dark. As they watched, a search-light leapt into being, and a pencil of light moved flickeringly across the sky. Then another and another--sweeping hither and thither like the blind feelers of some hidden octopus seeking its prey. There was something horribly uncanny in those long, straight shafts of light wavering uncertainly across the dense darkness of the night sky.

"Can you see the Zepp?" demanded Tim, with lively interest, from his bed.

"No, it's pitch black--too dark to see a thing," replied Sara.

Exactly as she spoke, a brilliant light hung for a moment suspended in the dark arch of the sky, then shivered into a blaze of garish effulgence, girdling the countryside and illuminating every road and building, every field, and tree, and ditch, as brightly as though it were broad daylight.

"A star-shell!" gasped Molly. "What a beastly thing! Positively"--giggling nervously--"I believe they can see right inside this room!"

"'Tisn't decent!" fulminated Jane indignantly, clutching with modest fingers at her scanty dressing-gown and straining it tightly across her chest whilst she backed hastily from the vicinity of the window. "Lightin' up sudden like that in the middle of the night! I feel for all the world as though I hadn't got a stitch on me! Come away from the window, do, miss----"

The light failed as suddenly as it had flared, and a warning crash, throbbing up against their ears, startled her into silence.

"That's a trifle too near to be pleasant," exclaimed Tim sharply. "Go downstairs, you three! Do you hear?"

Simultaneously, Selwyn shouted from below--

"Come downstairs! Come down at once! Quick, Sara! I'm coming up to carry Tim down--and Minnie won't stay alone. Come ***on***!"

Obedient to something urgent and imperative in the voices of both men--something that breathed of danger--the three women hastened from the room. Jane's candle flared and went out in the draught from the suddenly opened door, and in the smothering darkness they stumbled pell-mell down the stairs.

A dim light burning in the hall showed them Mrs. Selwyn cowering against her husband, her face hidden, sobbing hysterically, and in a moment Sara had taken Dick's place, wrapping her strong arms about the shuddering woman.

"Go on!" she whispered to him. "Go and get Tim down!"

He nodded, releasing himself with gentle force from his wife's clinging fingers, which had closed upon his arm like a vise.

Immediately she lifted up her voice in a thin, querulous shriek--

"No! Dick, Dick--don't leave me! ***Dick***"--

. . . And then it came--sped from that hovering Hate which hung above--dropping soundlessly, implacable through the utter darkness of the night and crashing into devilish life against a corner of the house.

Followed by a terrible flash and roar--a chaos of unimaginable sound. It seemed as though the whole world had split into fragments and were rocketing off into space; and, in quick succession, came the rumble of falling beams and masonry, and the dense dust of disintegrated plaster mingling with the fumes of high explosive.

Sara was conscious of being shot violently across the hall, and then everything went out in illimitable black darkness.

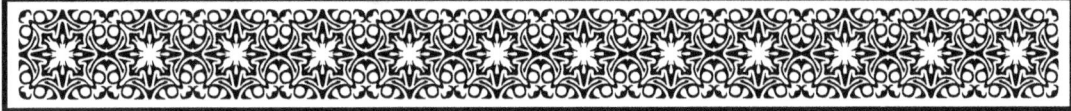

CHAPTER XXXVI
"FROM SUDDEN DEATH----"

S ara! Sara! For God's sake, open your eyes!"

The anguished tones pierced through the black curtain which had suddenly cut away the outer world from Sara's consciousness, and she opened her eyes obediently, to find herself looking straight into Garth's face bent above her--a sickly white in the yellow glare of the hurricane lamp he was holding.

"Are you hurt?" His voice came again insistently, sharp with hideous fear.

She sat up, breathing rather fast.

"No," she said, as though surprised. "I'm not hurt--not the least bit."

With Garth's help, she struggled to her feet and stood upright--rather shakily, it is true, but still able to accomplish the feat without much difficulty. She began to laugh weakly--a little helplessly.

"I think--I think I've only had my wind knocked out," she said. Then, as gradually the comprehension of events returned to her: "The others? Who's hurt? Oh, Garth! Is any one--*killed*?"

"No, no one, thank God!" He reassured her hastily. His arm went round her, and for a moment their lips met in a silent passion of thanksgiving.

"But you--how did you come here?" she asked, as they drew apart once more. "You . . . weren't . . . here?"--her brows contracting in a puzzled frown as she endeavoured to recall the incidents immediately preceding the bombing of the house. "We'd--we'd just gone to bed."

"I was dining with the Herricks. The raid began just as I was leaving them, so Judson and I drove straight on here instead of going home."

Sara pressed his hand.

"Bless you, dear!" she whispered quickly. Then, recollection returning more completely: "Tim? Is Tim safe?"

"Tim?"--sharply.

"He was upstairs. Where is Doctor Dick? Did he--"

"I'm not far off," came Selwyn's voice, from the mouth of a dark cavity that had once been the study doorway. "Come over here--but step carefully. The floor's strewn with stuff."

Garth piloted Sara skillfully across the debris that littered the floor, and they joined the group of shadowy figures huddled together in the doorless study.

"'Ware my arm!" warned Selwyn, as they approached. "It's broken, confound it!" He seemed, for the moment, oblivious of the pain.

Meanwhile, Mrs. Selwyn, finding herself physically intact, was keeping up an irritating moaning, interspersed with pettish diatribes against a Government that could be so culpably careless as to permit her to be bombed out of house and home; whilst Jane Crab, who had found and lit a candle, and recklessly stuck it to the table in its own grease, was bluffly endeavouring to console her.

For once Selwyn's saint-like patience failed him.

"Oh, shut up whining, Minnie!" he exclaimed forcefully. "It would be more to the point if you got down on your knees and said thank you to some one or something instead of grousing like that!"

He turned hurriedly to Garth, who was flashing his lantern hither and thither, locating the damage done.

"Look here," he said. "Young Durward's upstairs. We must get him down."

"Where does he sleep? One side of the house is staved in."

"He's not that side, thank Heaven! But the odds are he's badly hurt. And, anyway, he's helpless. I was just going up to carry him down when that damned bomb got us."

Garth swung out into the hall and sent a ringing shout up through the house. An instant later Tim's answer floated down to them.

"All serene! Can't move!"

Again Garth sent his voice pealing upwards--

"Hold on! We'll be with you in a minute."

He turned to Selwyn.

"I'll go up," he said. "You can't do anything with that arm of yours."

"I can help," maintained Dick stoutly.

Garth shook his head.

"No. If you slipped amongst the mess there'll be up there, I'd have two cripples on my hands instead of one. You stay here and look after the women--and get one of them to fix you up a temporary splint."

The two men moved forward, the women pressing eagerly behind them; then, as the light from Garth's lantern steamed ahead there came an instantaneous outcry of dismay.

The whole stairway was twisted and askew. It had a ludicrously drunken look, as though it were lolling up against the wall--like a staircase in a picture of which the perspective is all wrong.

"It isn't safe!" exclaimed Selwyn quickly. "You can't go up. We shall have to wait till help comes."

"I'm going up--now," said Garth quietly.

"But it isn't safe, man! Those stairs won't bear you!"

"They'll have to"--laconically. "That top story may go at any minute. It would collapse like a pack of cards if another bomb fell near enough for us to feel the concussion. And young Durward would have about as much chance as a rat in a trap."

A silence descended on the little group of anxious people as he finished speaking. The gravity of Tim's position suddenly revealed itself--and the danger involved by an attempt at rescue.

Sara drew close to Garth's side.

"*Must* you go, Garth?" she asked. "Wouldn't it be safe to wait till help comes?"

"Tim isn't *safe* there, actually five minutes. The floors may hold--or they mayn't! I must go, sweet."

She caught his hand and held it an instant against her cheek. Then--

"Go, dear," she whispered. "Go quickly. And oh!--God keep you!"

He was gone, picking his way gingerly, treading as lightly as a cat, so that the wrenched stairway hardly creaked beneath his swift, lithe steps.

Once there came the sudden rattle of some falling scrap of broken plaster, and Sara, leaning with closed eyes and white, set face, against the framework of a doorway, shivered soundlessly.

Soon he had disappeared round the distorted head of the staircase, and those who were watching could only discern the bobbing glimmer of the light he carried mounting higher and higher.

Then--after an interminable time, it seemed--there came the sound of voices . . . he had found Tim . . . a pause . . . then again a short, quick speech and the word "Right?" drifted faintly down to the strained ears below.

Unconsciously Sara's hands had clenched themselves, and the nails were biting into the flesh of her palms. But she felt no pain. Her whole being seemed concentrated into the single sense of hearing as she waited there in the candle-lit gloom, listening for every tiny sound, each creak of a board, each scattering of loosened plaster, which might herald danger.

Another eternity crawled by before, at length, Garth reappeared once more round the last bend of the staircase. Tim was lying across his shoulder, his injured leg hanging stiffly down, and in his hand he grasped the lantern, while both Garth's arms supported him.

Sara's eyes had opened now and fixed themselves intently on the burdened figure of the man she loved, as, with infinite caution, he began the descent of the last flight of stairs.

There was a double strain now upon the dislocated boards and joists--the weight of two men where one had climbed before with lithe, light, unimpeded limbs--and it seemed to Sara's tense, set vision as if a slight tremor ran throughout the whole stairway.

In an agony of terror she watched Garth's steady, downward progress. She felt as though she must scream out to him to hurry--*hurry*! Yet she bit back the scream lest it should startle him, every muscle of her body rigid with the effort that her silence cost her.

Seven stairs more! Six!

Sara's lips were moving voicelessly. She was whispering rapidly over and over again--

"God! God! God! Keep him safe! . . . You can do it. . . . Don't let him fall. . . ."

Five! Only five steps more!

"Hold up the stairs! . . . God! ***Don't*** let them give way! . . . Don't----"

Again there came the familiar thudding sound of an explosion. Somewhere another bomb, hurled from the cavernous dark that hid the enemy, had fallen, and almost simultaneously, it seemed, a warning thunder rumbled overhead like the menacing growl of a wild beast suddenly let loose.

At the first low mutter of that threat of imminent disaster, Garth sprang.

Gripping Tim firmly in his arms, he leaped from the quaking staircase, falling awkwardly, prone beneath the burden of the other's helpless body, as he landed.

And even as he reached the ground, the upper story of the house, with a roar that shook the whole remaining fabric of the building, crashed to earth in an avalanche of stone and brick and flying slates, whilst the stairway upon which he had been standing gave a sickening lurch, rocked, and fell out sideways into the hall in a smother of dust and plaster.

Stumblingly, those who had been watching groped their way through the powdery cloud, as it swirled and eddied, towards the dark blotch at the foot of the stairs which was all that could be distinguished of Trent and his burden.

To Sara, the momentary silence that ensued was in infinity of nameless dread. Then--

"We're all right," gasped Trent reassuringly, and choked violently as he inhaled a mouthful of grit-laden air.

In the same instant, across the murk shot a broad beam of light from the open doorway. Behind it Sara could discern white faces peering anxiously--Audrey's and Miles's, and, behind them again, loomed the heads and shoulders of others who had hurried to the scene of the catastrophe.

Then Herrick's voice rang out, high-pitched with gathering apprehension.

"Are you all safe?"

And when the reassuring answer reached the little throng upon the threshold, a murmur of relief went up, culminating in a ringing cheer as the news percolated through to the crowd which had collected in the roadway.

In an amazingly short time, so it seemed to Sara, she found herself comfortably tucked into the back seat of Garth's car, between him and Molly. Judson, with Jane beside him, took the wheel, and they were soon speeding swiftly away towards Greenacres, where Audrey had insisted that the homeless household must take refuge--the remainder of the party following in the Herricks' limousine.

It had been a night of adventure, but it was over at last, and, as Jane Crab remarked with stolid conviction--

"The doctor--blessed saint!--was never intended to be killed by one of they 'Uns, so they might as well have saved theirselves the trouble of trying it--and we'd all have slept the easier in our beds!"

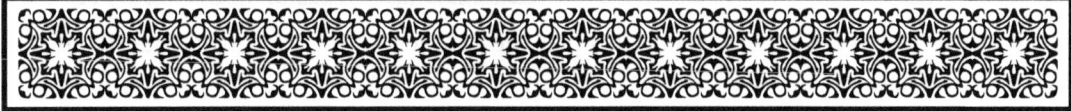

CHAPTER XXXVII
THE RECKONING

Elisabeth came slowly out of the room where her son was lying. She had reached Greenacres--in response to Sara's letter, posted on the eve of the raid--late in the afternoon of the following day, and Audrey had at once taken her upstairs to see Tim and left them together. And now, as she closed the door of his room behind her, she leaned helplessly against the wall and her lips moved in a whispered cry of poignant misery.

"Maurice! . . . Maurice saved him! . . . Oh, my God!"

Her eyes--the beautiful, hyacinth eyes--stared strickenly in front of her, wide and horrified like the eyes of a hunted thing, and her hands were twisted and wrung beneath the stress of the overwhelming knowledge which Tim had so joyously prattled out to her. She could hear him now, boyishly enthusiastic, extolling Garth with the eager, unstinted hero-worship of youth, and every word he said had pierced her like the stab of a knife.

"If ever a chap deserved the V.C., Trent does, by Jove! It was the bravest thing I've ever known, mother mine, for he told me afterwards, he never expected that the top story would hold out till he got me away. He'd seen it from the outside first, you know! And there was I, held up with this confounded ankle, **and** with a whole heap of plaster and a brick or two sitting on my chest I thought I'd gone west that time, for a certainty!"

And Tim chuckled delightedly, blissfully unconscious that with each word he spoke he was binding upon his mother's shoulders an insuperable burden of remorse.

It was Garth Trent who had saved her son--Garth Trent, to whom she owed all the garnered happiness of her married life, yet whose own life's fabric she had pulled down about his ears! And now, to the already overwhelming magnitude of her debt to him, he had added this--this final act of sacrifice.

With an almost superhuman effort, Elisabeth had forced herself to listen quietly to Tim's account of his rescue from the shattered upper story of the Selwyn's house--to listen precisely as though Garth's share in the matter held no particular significance for her beyond the splendid one it must inevitably hold for any mother.

But now, safe from the clear-sighted glance of Tim's blue eyes, she let the mask slip from her and crouched against his door in uncontrollable agony of spirit.

The sin which she had sinned in secret--which, sometimes, she had almost come to believe was not a sin, so beautiful had been its fruit--revealed itself to her now in all its naked ugliness.

Looking backward, down the vista of years, the whole structure of her happiness appeared in its true perspective, reared upon a lie--upon that same lie which had blasted Garth Trent's career and sent him out, dishonoured, from the company of his fellows.

And this man from whom she had taken faith, and hope, and good repute--everything, in fact, that makes a man's life worth having--had given her the life of her son!

She dropped her face between her hands with a low moan. It was horrible--horrible.

Then, afraid that Tim might hear her, she passed stumblingly into her own room at the end of the corridor, and there, in solitude and darkness, she fought out the battle between her desire still to preserve the secret she had guarded three-and-twenty years, and the impulse toward atonement which was struggling into life within her.

Like a scourge the knowledge of her debt to Garth drove her before it, beating her into the very depths of self-abasement, but, even so, her pride of name, and the mother-love which yearned to shield her son from all that it must involve if she should now confess the sin of her youth, urged her to let the present still keep the secrets of the past.

The habit of years, the very purpose for which she had worked, and lied, and fought, must be renounced if she were to make atonement. A tale that was unbelievably shameful must be revealed--and Tim would have to know all that there was to be known.

To Elisabeth, this was the most bitter thing she had to face--the fact that Tim, for whose sake she had so strenuously guarded her secret, must learn, not only what was written on that turned-down page of life, but also what kind of woman his mother had proved herself--how totally unlike the beautiful conception which his ardent boyish faith in her had formed.

Would he understand? Would he ever understand--and forgive?

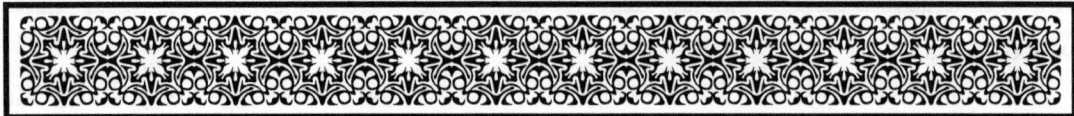

CHAPTER XXXVIII
VINDICATION

Meanwhile, the Herricks and their guests--"Audrey's refugees," as Molly elected to describe the latter, herself included--had gathered round the fire in the library, and were chatting desultorily while they awaited Elisabeth's return from her visit to Tim's sick-room.

The casualties of the previous evening had been found to be augmented by two, since Mrs. Selwyn had remained in bed throughout the day, under the impression that she was suffering from shock, whilst Garth Trent was discovered to have dislocated his shoulder, and had been compelled to keep his room by medical orders.

In endeavouring to shield Tim, as they crashed to the ground together from the tottering staircase, Trent had fallen undermost, receiving the full brunt of the fall; and a dislocated shoulder and a severe shaking, which had left him bruised and sore from head to foot, were the consequences.

Characteristically, he had maintained complete silence about his injury, composedly accompanying Sara back to Greenacres in his car, and he had just been making his way out of the house when he had quietly fainted away on to the floor. After which, the Herricks had taken over command.

"I think," remarked Molly pertinently, "you might as well turn Greenacres into an annexe to the 'Convalescent,' Audrey. You've got four cases already."

The Lavender Lady glanced up smilingly from one of the khaki socks which, in these days, dangled perpetually from her shining needles, and into which she knitted all the love, and pity, and tender prayers of her simple old heart.

"Mr. Trent is better," she announced with satisfaction. "I had tea upstairs with him this afternoon."

"Yes," supplements Selwyn, "I fancy one of your patients has struck, Audrey.

Trent intends coming down this evening. Judson has just come back from Far End with some fresh clothes for him."

Audrey turned hastily to her husband.

"Good Heavens, Miles! We can't let him come down! Mrs. Durward will be here with us."

"Well?"--placidly from Herrick.

"Well! It will be anything but well!" retorted Audrey significantly. "Have you forgotten what happened that day in Haven Woods? I'm not going to have Garth hurt like that again! He may have been cashiered a hundred times--I don't care whether he was or not!--he's a man!"

A very charming smile broke over Miles's face.

"I've always known it," he said quietly. "And--I should think Mrs. Durward knows it now."

"Yes. I know it now."

The low, contralto tones that answered were Elisabeth's. Unnoticed, she had entered the room and was standing just outside the little group of people clustered round the hearth--her slim, black-robed figure, with its characteristic little air of stateliness, sharply defined in the ruddy glow of the firelight.

A sudden tremor of emotion seemed to ripple through the room. The atmosphere grew tense, electric--alert as with some premonition of coming storm.

The two men had risen to their feet, but no one spoke, and the brief rustle of movement, as every one turned instinctively towards that slender, sable figure, whispered into blank silence.

To Miles, infinitely compassionate, there seemed something symbolical in the figure of the woman standing there--isolated, outside the friendly circle of the fireside group, standing solitary at the table as a prisoner stands at the bar of judgment.

The firelight, flickering across her face, revealed its pallor and the burning fever of her eyes, and drew strange lights from the heavy chestnut hair that swathed her head like a folded banner of flame.

For a long moment she stood silently regarding the ring of startled faces turned towards her. Then at last she spoke.

"I have something to tell you," she said, addressing herself primarily, it seemed, to Miles.

Perhaps she recognized the compassionate spirit of understanding which was his in so great a measure and appealed to it unconsciously. Selwyn, with sensitive perception, turned as though to leave the room, but she stopped him.

"No, don't go," she said quickly. "Please stay--all of you. I--I wish you all to hear what I have to say." She spoke very composedly, with a curious submissive dignity, as though she had schooled herself to meet this moment. "It concerns Garth Trent--at least, that is the name by which you know him. His real name is Maurice--Maurice Kennedy, and he is my cousin, Lord Grisdale's younger son. He has lived here under an assumed name because--because"--her voice trembled a little, then steadied again to its accustomed even quality--"because I ruined his life. . . . The only way in which I can make amends is by telling you the true facts of the Indian Frontier episode which led to Maurice's dismissal from the Army. He--ought never to have been--cashiered for cowardice."

She paused, and with a sudden instinctive movement Sara grasped Selwyn's arm, while the sharp sibilance of her quick-drawn breath cut across the momentary silence.

"No," Elisabeth repeated. "Maurice ought never to have been cashiered. He was absolutely innocent of the charge against him. The real offender was Geoffrey . . . my husband. It was he--Geoffrey, not Maurice--who was sent out in charge of the reconnaissance party from the fort--and it was he whose nerve gave way when surprised by the enemy. Maurice kept his head and tried to steady him, but, at the time, Geoffrey must have been mad--caught by sudden panic, together with his men. Don't judge him too hardly"--her voice took on a note of pleading--"you must remember that he had been enduring days and nights of frightful strain, and that the attack came without any warning . . . in the darkness. He had no time to think--to pull himself together. And he lost his head. . . . Maurice did his best to save the situation. Realizing that for the moment Geoffrey was hardly accountable, he deliberately shot him in the leg, to incapacitate him, and took command himself, trying to rally the men. But they stampeded past him, panic-stricken, and it was while he was storming at them to turn round and put up a fight that--that he was shot in the back." She faltered, meeting the measureless reproach in Sara's eyes, and strickenly aware of the hateful interpretation she had put upon the same incident when describing it to her on a former occasion.

For the first time, she seemed to lose her composure, rocking a little where she stood and supporting herself by gripping the edge of the table with straining fingers.

But no one stirred. In poignant silence they awaited the continuance of the tale which each one sensed to be developing towards a climax of inevitable calamity.

"Afterwards," pursued Elisabeth at last, "at the court-martial, two of the men gave evidence that they had seen Geoffrey fall wounded at the beginning of the skirmish--they did not know that it was Maurice who had disabled him intentionally--so that he was completely exonerated from all blame, and the Court came to the conclusion that, the command having thus fallen to Maurice, he had lost his nerve and been guilty of cowardice in face of the enemy. Geoffrey himself knew nothing of the actual facts--either then or later. He had gone down like a log when Maurice shot him, striking his head as he fell, and concussion of the brain wiped out of his mind all recollection of what had occurred in the fight prior to his fall. The last thing he remembered was mustering his men together in readiness to leave the fort. Everything else was a blank."

Out of the shadows of the fire-lit room came a muttered question.

"Yes." Elisabeth bent her head in answer. "There was--other evidence forthcoming. But not then, not at the time of the trial. Then Maurice was dismissed from the Army."

She seemed to speak with ever-increasing difficulty, and her hand went up suddenly to her throat. It was obvious that this self-imposed disclosure of the truth was taking her strength to its uttermost limit.

"I had better tell you the whole story--from the beginning," she said, at last, haltingly, and, after a moment's hesitation, she resumed in the hard, expressionless voice of intense effort.

"Before Maurice went out to India, he and I were engaged to be married. On my part, it would have been only a marriage of convenience, for I was not in love with him, although I had always been fond of him in a cousinly way. There was another man whom I loved--the man I afterwards married, Geoffrey Lovell--" for an instant her eyes glowed with a sudden radiance of remembrance--"and he and I became secretly engaged, in spite of the fact that I had already promised to marry Maurice. I expect you think that was unforgivable of me," she seemed to search the intent faces of her little audience as though challenging the verdict she might read therein; "but there was some excuse. I was very young, and at the time I promised myself to Maurice I did not know that Geoffrey cared for me. And then--when I knew--I hadn't the courage to break with Maurice. He and Geoffrey were both going out to India--they were in the same regiment--and I kept hoping that something might happen which would make it easier for me. Maurice might meet and be attracted by some other woman. . . . I hoped he would."

She fell silent for a moment, then, gathering her remaining strength together, as it seemed, she went on relentlessly--

"Something did happen. Maurice was cashiered from the Army, and I had a legitimate reason for terminating the engagement between us. . . . Then, just as I thought I was free, he came to tell me his case would be reopened; there was an eye-witness who could prove his innocence, a private in his own regiment. I never knew who the man was"--she turned slightly at the sound of a sudden brusque movement from Miles Herrick, then, as he volunteered no remark, continued--"but it appeared he had been badly wounded and had only learned the verdict of the court-martial after his recovery. He had then written to Maurice, telling him that he was in a position to prove that it was not he, but Geoffrey Lovell who had been guilty of cowardice. When I understood this, and realized what it must mean, I confessed to Maurice that Geoffrey was the man I loved, and I begged and implored him to take the blame--to let the verdict of the court-marital stand. It was a horrible thing to do--I know that . . . but think what it meant to me! It meant the honour and welfare of the man I loved, as opposed to the honour and welfare of a man for whom I cared comparatively little. Maurice was not easy to move, but I made him understand that, whatever happened now, I should never marry him--that I should sink or swim with Geoffrey, and at last he consented to do the thing I asked. He accepted the blame and went away--to the Colonies, I believe. Afterwards, as you all know, he returned to England and lived at Far End under the name of Garth Trent."

Such was the tale Elisabeth unfolded, and the hushed listeners, keyed up by its tragic drama, could visualize for themselves the scene of that last piteous interview between Elisabeth and the man who had loved her to his own utter undoing.

She was still a very lovely woman, and it was easy to realize how well-nigh bewilderingly beautiful she must have been in her youth, easy to imagine how Garth--or Maurice Kennedy, as he must henceforth be recognized--worshipping her with a boy's headlong passion, had agreed to let the judgment of the Court remain unchallenged and to shoulder the burden of another man's sin.

Probably he felt that, since he had lost her, nothing else mattered, and, with the reckless chivalry of youth, he never stopped to count the cost. He only knew that the woman he loved, whose beauty pierced him to the very soul, so that his vision was blurred by the sheer loveliness of her, demanded her happiness at his hands and that he must give it to her.

"I suppose you think there was no excuse for what I did," Elisabeth concluded, with something of appeal in her voice. "But I did not realize, then, quite all that I was taking from Maurice. I think that much must be granted me. . . . But I make no excuse for what I did afterwards. There is none. I did it deliberately. Maurice had won the woman Tim wanted, and I hoped that if he were utterly discredited, Sara would refuse to marry him, and thus the way would be open to Tim. So I made public the story of the court-martial which had sentenced Maurice. Had it not been for that, I should have held my peace for ever about his having been cashiered. I--I owed him that much." She was silent a moment. Presently she raised her head and spoke in harsh, wrung accents. "But I've been punished! God saw to that. What do you think it has meant to me to know that my husband--the man I worshipped-- had been once a coward? It's true the world never knew it . . . but I knew it."

The agony of pride wounded in its most sacred place, the suffering of love that despises what it loves, yet cannot cease from loving, rang in her voice, and her haunted eyes--the eyes which had guarded their secret so invincibly--seemed to plead for comfort, for understanding.

It was Miles who answered that unspoken supplication.

"I think you need never feel shame again," he said very gently. "Major Durward's splendid death has more than wiped out that one mistake of his youth. Thank God he never knew it needed wiping out."

A momentary tranquility came into Elisabeth's face.

"No," she answered simply. "No, he never knew." Then the tide of bitter recollection surged over her once more, and she continued passionately: "Oh yes, I've been punished! Day and night, day and night since the war began, I've lived in terror that the fear--his father's fear--might suddenly grip Tim out there in Flanders. I kept him out of the Army--because I was afraid. And then the war came, and he had to go. Thank God--oh, thank God!--he never failed! . . . I suppose I am a bad woman--I don't know . . . I fought for my own love and happiness first, and afterwards for my son's. But, at least, I'm not bad enough to let Maurice go on bearing . . . what he has borne . . . now that he has saved Tim's life. He has given me the only thing . . . left to me . . . of value in the whole world. In return, I can give him the one thing that matters to him--his good name. Henceforth Maurice is a free man."

" *What* are you saying?"

The sharp, staccato question cut across Elisabeth's quiet, concentrated speech like a rapier thrust, snapping the strained attention of her listeners, who turned, with one accord, to see Kennedy himself standing at the threshold of the room, his eyes fastened on Elisabeth's face.

She met his glance composedly; on her lips a queer little smile which held an indefinable pathos and appeal.

"I am telling them the truth--at last, Maurice," she said calmly. "I have told them the true story of the court-martial."

"You--you have told them *that*?" he stammered. He was very pale. The sudden realization of all that her words implied seemed to overwhelm him.

"Yes." She rose and moved quietly to the door, then face to face with Kennedy, she halted. Her eyes rested levelly on his; in her bearing there was something aloofly proud--an undiminished stateliness, almost regal in its calm inviolability. "They know--now--all that I took from you. I shall not ask your forgiveness, Maurice . . . I don't expect it. I sinned for my husband and my son--that is my only justification. I would do the same again."

Instinctively Maurice stood aside as she swept past him, her head unbowed, splendid even in her moment of surrender--almost, it seemed, unbeaten to the last.

For a moment there was a silence--palpitant, packed with conflicting emotion.

Then, with a little choking sob, Sara ran across the room to Maurice and caught his hands in hers, smiling whilst the tears streamed down her cheeks.

"Oh, my dear!" she cried brokenly. "Oh, my dear!"

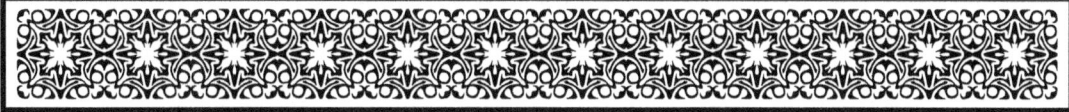

CHAPTER XXXIX
HARVEST

"There shall never be one lost good! What was, shall live
as before;
The evil is null, is nought, is silence implying sound;
What was good, shall be good, with, for evil,
So much good more . . ."
BROWNING.

How can you prove it, Garth--Maurice, I mean?"--Selwyn corrected himself with a smile. "You'll need more than Mrs. Durward's confession to secure official reinstatement by the powers that be."

The clamour of joyful excitement and wonder and congratulation had spent itself at last, the Lavender Lady had shed a few legitimate tears, and now Selwyn voiced the more serious aspect of the matter.

It was Herrick who made answer.

"I have the necessary proofs," he said quietly. He had crossed to a bureau in the corner of the room, and now returned with a packet of papers in his hand.

"These," he pursued, "are from my brother Colin, who is farming in Australia. He was a good many years my senior--and I've always understood that he was a bit of a ne'er-do-well in his younger days. Ultimately, he enlisted in the Army as a Tommy, and in that scrap on the Indian Frontier he was close behind Maurice and saw the whole thing. He got badly wounded then, and was dangerously ill for some time afterwards, so it happened that he knew nothing about the court-martial till it was all over. When he recovered, he wrote to Maurice, offering his evidence, and"--smiling whimsically across at Kennedy--"received a haughty letter in reply, assuring him that he was mistaken in the facts and that the writer did not dispute the verdict of the court. My brother rather suspected some wild-cat business, so before he went to Australia, some years later, he placed in my hands properly witnessed documents containing the true facts of the matter, and it was only when, through Mrs. Durward, we learned that Maurice had been cashiered from the Army, that the connection between that and the Frontier incident flashed into my mind as a possibility. I had heard that the Durwards' name had been originally Lovell—and I began to wonder if Garth Trent's name had not been originally"—with a glint of humour in his eyes—"Maurice Kennedy! Here's my brother's letter"—passing it to Sara, who was standing next him—"and here's the document which he left in my care. I've had 'em both locked away since I was seventeen."

Sara's eyes flew down the few brief lines of the letter.

"Evidently the young fool wishes to be thought guilty," Colin Herrick had written. "Shielding his pal Lovell, I suppose. Well, it's his funeral, not mine! But one never knows how things may pan out, and some day it might mean all the difference between heaven and hell to Kennedy to be able to prove his innocence—so I am enclosing herewith a properly attested record of the facts, Miles, in case I should send in my checks while I'm at the other side of the world."

As a matter of fact, however, Colin still lived and prospered in Australia, so that there would be no difficulty in proving Maurice's innocence down to the last detail.

"Do you mean," Sara appealed to Miles incredulously, "do you mean—that there were these proofs—all the time? And you—*you knew*?"

"Herrick wasn't to blame," interposed Maurice hastily, sensing the horrified accusation in her tones. "I forbade him to use those papers."

"But why—why———"

Miles looked at her and a light kindled in his eyes.

"My dear, you're marrying a chivalrous, quixotic fool. Maurice refused to let me show these proofs because, on the strength of his promise to shield Geoffrey Lovell, Elisabeth had married and borne a son. Not even though it meant smashing up his whole life would he go back on his word."

"Garth! Garth!" The name by which she had always known him sprang spontaneously from Sara's lips. Her voice was shaking, but her eyes, likes Herrick's, held a glory of quiet shining. "How could you, dear? What madness! What idiotic, glorious madness!"

"I don't see how I could have done anything else," said Maurice simply. "Elisabeth's whole scheme of existence was fashioned on her trust in my promise. I couldn't--afterwards, after her marriage and Tim's birth--suddenly pull away the very foundation on which she had built up her life."

Impulsively Sara slipped her hand into his.

"I'm glad--*glad* you couldn't, dear," she whispered. "It would not have been my Garth if you could have done."

He pressed her hand in silence. A curious lassitude was stealing over him. He had borne the heat and burden of the day, and now that the work was done and there was nothing further to fight for, nothing left to struggle and contend against, he was conscious of a strange feeling of frustration.

It seemed almost as though the long agony of those years of self-immolation had been in vain--a useless sacrifice, made meaningless and of no account by the destined march of events.

He felt vaguely baulked and disillusioned--bewildered that a man's aim and purpose, which in its accomplishing had cost so immeasurable a price--crushing the whole beauty and savour out of life--should suddenly be destroyed and nullified. In the light of the present, the past seemed futile--years that the locust had eaten.

It was a relief when presently some one broke in upon the confused turmoil of his thoughts with a message from Tim. He was asking to see both Sara and Maurice--would they go to him?

Together they went up to his room--Maurice still with that look of grave perplexity upon his face which his somewhat bitter reflections had engendered.

The eager, boyish face on the pillow flushed a little as they entered.

"Mother has told me everything," he said simply, going straight to the point. "It's--it's been rather a facer."

Maurice pointed to the narrow ribbon--the white, purple, white of the Military Cross--upon the breast of the khaki tunic flung across a chair-back--a rather disheveled tunic, rescued with other odds and ends from the wreckage of Tim's room at Sunnyside.

"It needn't be, Tim," he said, "with that to your credit."

Tim's eyes glowed.

"That's just it--that's what I wanted to see you for," he said. "I hope you won't think it cheek," he went on rather shyly, "but I wanted you to know that--that what you did for my mother--assuming the disgrace, I mean, that wasn't yours-- hasn't been all wasted. What little I've done--well, it would never have been done had I known what I know now."

"I think it would," Maurice dissented quietly.

Tim shook his head.

"No. Had my father been cashiered--for cowardice"--he stumbled a little over the words--"the knowledge of it would have knocked all the initiative out of me. I should have been afraid of showing the white feather. . . . The fear of being afraid would have been always at the back of me." He paused, then went on quickly: "And I think it would have been the same with Dad. It--it would have broken him. He could never have fought as he did with that behind him. You've . . . you've given two men to the country. . . ."

He broke off, boyishly embarrassed, a little overwhelmed by his own big thoughts.

And suddenly to Maurice, all that had been dark and obscure grew clear in the white shining of the light that gleamed down the track of those lost years.

A beautiful and ordered issue was revealed. Out of the ruin and bleak suffering of the past had sprung the flaming splendour of heroic life and death--a glory of achievement that, but for those arid years of silence, had been thwarted and frustrated by the deadening knowledge of the truth.

Kindling to the recognition of new and wonderful significances, his eyes sought those of the woman who loved him, and in their quiet radiance he read that she, too, had understood.

For her, as for him, the dark places had been made light, and with quickened vision she perceived, in all that had befallen, the fulfilling of the Divine law.

"Sara----"

Her hands went out to him, and the grave happiness deepened in her eyes.

"Oh, my dear, no love--no sacrifice is ever wasted!"

She spoke very simply, very confidently.

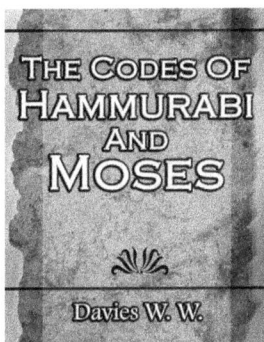

The Codes Of Hammurabi And Moses
W. W. Davies

QTY

The discovery of the Hammurabi Code is one of the greatest achievements of archaeology, and is of paramount interest, not only to the student of the Bible, but also to all those interested in ancient history...

Religion   **ISBN: *1-59462-338-4***   **Pages:132**
                                                    MSRP $12.95

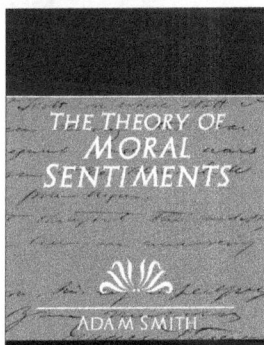

The Theory of Moral Sentiments
Adam Smith

QTY

This work from 1749. contains original theories of conscience amd moral judgment and it is the foundation for systemof morals.

Philosophy   ISBN: *1-59462-777-0*   **Pages:536**
                                                MSRP $19.95

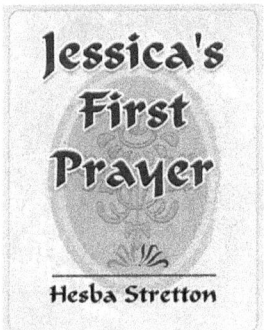

Jessica's First Prayer
Hesba Stretton

QTY

In a screened and secluded corner of one of the many railway-bridges which span the streets of London there could be seen a few years ago, from five o'clock every morning until half past eight, a tidily set-out coffee-stall, consisting of a trestle and board, upon which stood two large tin cans, with a small fire of charcoal burning under each so as to keep the coffee boiling during the early hours of the morning when the work-people were thronging into the city on their way to their daily toil...

Pages:84

Childrens   ISBN: *1-59462-373-2*   *MSRP $9.95*

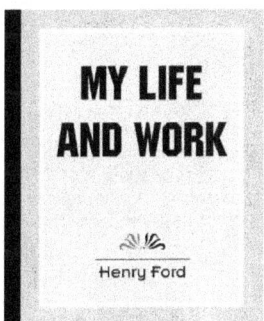

My Life and Work
Henry Ford

QTY

Henry Ford revolutionized the world with his implementation of mass production for the Model T automobile. Gain valuable business insight into his life and work with his own auto-biography... "We have only started on our development of our country we have not as yet, with all our talk of wonderful progress, done more than scratch the surface. The progress has been wonderful enough but..."

Pages:300

Biographies/   ISBN: *1-59462-198-5*   *MSRP $21.95*

www.bookjungle.com *email: sales@bookjungle.com fax: 630-214-0564 mail: Book Jungle PO Box 2226 Champaign, IL 61825*

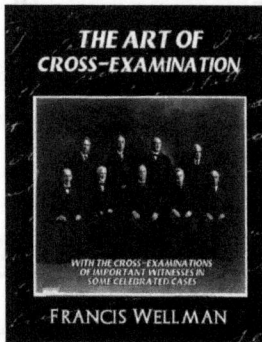

The Art of Cross-Examination
Francis Wellman

QTY

I presume it is the experience of every author, after his first book is published upon an important subject, to be almost overwhelmed with a wealth of ideas and illustrations which could readily have been included in his book, and which to his own mind, at least, seem to make a second edition inevitable. Such certainly was the case with me; and when the first edition had reached its sixth impression in five months, I rejoiced to learn that it seemed to my publishers that the book had met with a sufficiently favorable reception to justify a second and considerably enlarged edition. ..

Pages:412

Reference   ISBN: *1-59462-647-2*   *MSRP $19.95*

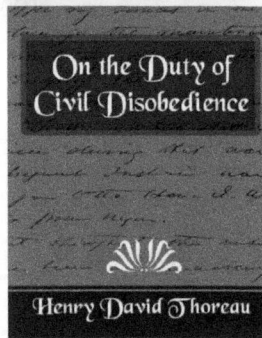

On the Duty of Civil Disobedience
Henry David Thoreau

QTY

Thoreau wrote his famous essay, On the Duty of Civil Disobedience, as a protest against an unjust but popular war and the immoral but popular institution of slave-owning. He did more than write—he declined to pay his taxes,   and was hauled off to gaol in consequence. Who can say how much this refusal of his hastened the end of the war and of slavery ?

Law   ISBN: *1-59462-747-9*   **Pages:48**

MSRP $7.45

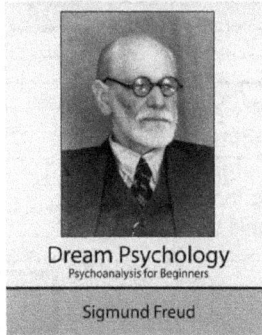

Dream Psychology Psychoanalysis for Beginners
Sigmund Freud

QTY

Sigmund Freud, born Sigismund Schlomo Freud (May 6, 1856 - September 23, 1939), was a Jewish-Austrian neurologist and psychiatrist who co-founded the psychoanalytic school of psychology. Freud is best known for his theories of the unconscious mind, especially involving the mechanism of repression; his redefinition of sexual desire as mobile and directed towards a wide variety of objects; and his therapeutic techniques, especially his understanding of transference in the therapeutic relationship and the presumed value of dreams as sources of insight into unconscious desires.

Pages:196

Psychology   ISBN: *1-59462-905-6*   *MSRP $15.45*

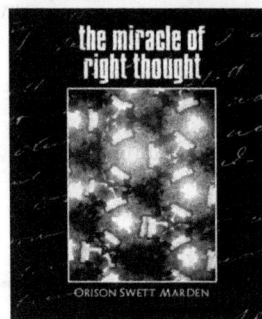

The Miracle of Right Thought
Orison Swett Marden

QTY

Believe with all of your heart that you will do what you were made to do. When the mind has once formed the habit of holding cheerful, happy, prosperous pictures, it will not be easy to form the opposite habit. It does not matter how improbable or how far away this realization may see, or how dark the prospects may be, if we visualize them as best we can, as vividly as possible, hold tenaciously to them and vigorously struggle to attain them, they will gradually become actualized, realized in the life. But a desire, a longing without endeavor, a yearning abandoned or held indifferently will vanish without realization.

Pages:360

Self Help   ISBN: *1-59462-644-8*   *MSRP $25.45*

QTY

The Rosicrucian Cosmo-Conception Mystic Christianity by *Max Heindel*   ISBN: *1-59462-188-8*   **$38.95**
The Rosicrucian Cosmo-conception is not dogmatic, neither does it appeal to any other authority than the reason of the student. It is: not controversial, but is: sent forth in the, hope that it may help to clear...   New Age/Religion Pages 646

Abandonment To Divine Providence by *Jean-Pierre de Caussade*   ISBN: *1-59462-228-0*   **$25.95**
"The Rev. Jean Pierre de Caussade was one of the most remarkable spiritual writers of the Society of Jesus in France in the 18th Century. His death took place at Toulouse in 1751. His works have gone through many editions and have been republished...   Inspirational/Religion Pages 400

Mental Chemistry by *Charles Haanel*   ISBN: *1-59462-192-6*   **$23.95**
Mental Chemistry allows the change of material conditions by combining and appropriately utilizing the power of the mind. Much like applied chemistry creates something new and unique out of careful combinations of chemicals the mastery of mental chemistry...   New Age/Business Pages 354

The Letters of Robert Browning and Elizabeth Barret Barrett 1845-1846 vol II   ISBN: *1-59462-193-4*   **$35.95**
by *Robert Browning* and *Elizabeth Barrett*   Biographies Pages 596

Gleanings In Genesis (volume I) by *Arthur W. Pink*   ISBN: *1-59462-130-6*   **$27.45**
Appropriately has Genesis been termed "the seed plot of the Bible" for in it we have, in germ form, almost all of the great doctrines which are afterwards fully developed in the books of Scripture which follow...   Religion/Inspirational Pages 420

The Master Key by *L. W. de Laurence*   ISBN: *1-59462-001-6*   **$30.95**
In no branch of human knowledge has there been a more lively increase of the spirit of research during the past few years than in the study of Psychology, Concentration and Mental Discipline. The requests for authentic lessons in Thought Control, Mental Discipline and...   New Age Pages 422

The Lesser Key Of Solomon Goetia by *L. W. de Laurence*   ISBN: *1-59462-092-X*   **$9.95**
This translation of the first book of the "Lernegton" which is now for the first time made accessible to students of Talismanic Magic was done, after careful collation and edition, from numerous Ancient Manuscripts in Hebrew, Latin, and French...   New Age/Occult Pages 92

Rubaiyat Of Omar Khayyam by *Edward Fitzgerald*   ISBN:*1-59462-332-5*   **$13.95**
Edward Fitzgerald, whom the world has already learned, in spite of his own efforts to remain within the shadow of anonymity, to look upon as one of the rarest poets of the century, was born at Bredfield, in Suffolk, on the 31st of March, 1809. He was the third son of John Purcell...   Music Pages 172

Ancient Law by *Henry Maine*   ISBN: *1-59462-128-4*   **$29.95**
The chief object of the following pages is to indicate some of the earliest ideas of mankind, as they are reflected in Ancient Law, and to point out the relation of those ideas to modern thought.   Religion/History Pages 452

Far-Away Stories by *William J. Locke*   ISBN: *1-59462-129-2*   **$19.45**
"Good wine needs no bush, but a collection of mixed vintages does. And this book is just such a collection. Some of the stories I do not want to remain buried for ever in the museum files of dead magazine-numbers an author's not unpardonable vanity..."   Fiction Pages 272

Life of David Crockett by *David Crockett*   ISBN: *1-59462-250-7*   **$27.45**
"Colonel David Crockett was one of the most remarkable men of the times in which he lived. Born in humble life, but gifted with a strong will, an indomitable courage, and unremitting perseverance...   Biographies/New Age Pages 424

Lip-Reading by *Edward Nitchie*   ISBN: *1-59462-206-X*   **$25.95**
Edward B. Nitchie, founder of the New York School for the Hard of Hearing, now the Nitchie School of Lip-Reading, Inc, wrote "LIP-READING Principles and Practice". The development and perfecting of this meritorious work on lip-reading was an undertaking...   How-to Pages 400

A Handbook of Suggestive Therapeutics, Applied Hypnotism, Psychic Science   ISBN: *1-59462-214-0*   **$24.95**
by *Henry Munro*   Health/New Age/Health/Self-help Pages 376

A Doll's House: and Two Other Plays by *Henrik Ibsen*   ISBN: *1-59462-112-8*   **$19.95**
Henrik Ibsen created this classic when in revolutionary 1848 Rome. Introducing some striking concepts in playwriting for the realist genre, this play has been studied the world over.   Fiction/Classics/Plays 308

The Light of Asia by *sir Edwin Arnold*   ISBN: *1-59462-204-3*   **$13.95**
In this poetic masterpiece, Edwin Arnold describes the life and teachings of Buddha. The man who was to become known as Buddha to the world was born as Prince Gautama of India but he rejected the worldly riches and abandoned the reigns of power when... Religion/History/Biographies Pages 170

The Complete Works of Guy de Maupassant by *Guy de Maupassant*   ISBN: *1-59462-157-8*   **$16.95**
"For days and days, nights and nights, I had dreamed of that first kiss which was to consecrate our engagement, and I knew not on what spot I should put my lips..."   Fiction/Classics Pages 240

The Art of Cross-Examination by *Francis L. Wellman*   ISBN: *1-59462-309-0*   **$26.95**
Written by a renowned trial lawyer, Wellman imparts his experience and uses case studies to explain how to use psychology to extract desired information through questioning.   How-to/Science/Reference Pages 408

Answered or Unanswered? by *Louisa Vaughan*   ISBN: *1-59462-248-5*   **$10.95**
Miracles of Faith in China   Religion Pages 112

The Edinburgh Lectures on Mental Science (1909) by *Thomas*   ISBN: *1-59462-008-3*   **$11.95**
This book contains the substance of a course of lectures recently given by the writer in the Queen Street Hall, Edinburgh. Its purpose is to indicate the Natural Principles governing the relation between Mental Action and Material Conditions...   New Age/Psychology Pages 148

Ayesha by *H. Rider Haggard*   ISBN: *1-59462-301-5*   **$24.95**
Verily and indeed it is the unexpected that happens! Probably if there was one person upon the earth from whom the Editor of this, and of a certain previous history, did not expect to hear again...   Classics Pages 380

Ayala's Angel by *Anthony Trollope*   ISBN: *1-59462-352-X*   **$29.95**
The two girls were both pretty, but Lucy who was twenty-one who supposed to be simple and comparatively unattractive, whereas Ayala was credited, as her Bombwhat romantic name might show, with poetic charm and a taste for romance. Ayala when her father died was nineteen...   Fiction Pages 484

The American Commonwealth by *James Bryce*   ISBN: *1-59462-286-8*   **$34.45**
An interpretation of American democratic political theory. It examines political mechanics and society from the perspective of Scotsman James Bryce   Politics Pages 572

Stories of the Pilgrims by *Margaret P. Pumphrey*   ISBN: *1-59462-116-0*   **$17.95**
This book explores pilgrims religious oppression in England as well as their escape to Holland and eventual crossing to America on the Mayflower, and their early days in New England...   History Pages 268

www.bookjungle.com *email: sales@bookjungle.com fax: 630-214-0564 mail: Book Jungle PO Box 2226 Champaign, IL 61825*

QTY

The Fasting Cure by *Sinclair Upton*   ISBN: *1-59462-222-1*   **$13.95**
*In the Cosmopolitan Magazine for May, 1910, and in the Contemporary Review (London) for April, 1910, I published an article dealing with my experi-
ences in fasting. I have written a great many magazine articles, but never one which attracted so much attention... New Age/Self Help/Health Pages 164*

Hebrew Astrology by *Sepharial*   ISBN: *1-59462-308-2*   **$13.45**
*In these days of advanced thinking it is a matter of common observation that we have left many of the old landmarks behind and that we are now pressing
forward to greater heights and to a wider horizon than that which represented the mind-content of our progenitors...   Astrology Pages 144*

Thought Vibration or The Law of Attraction in the Thought World   ISBN: *1-59462-127-6*   **$12.95**
by *William Walker Atkinson*   *Psychology/Religion Pages 144*

Optimism by *Helen Keller*   ISBN: *1-59462-108-X*   **$15.95**
*Helen Keller was blind, deaf, and mute since 19 months old, yet famously learned how to overcome these handicaps, communicate with the world, and
spread her lectures promoting optimism. An inspiring read for everyone...   Biographies/Inspirational Pages 84*

Sara Crewe by *Frances Burnett*   ISBN: *1-59462-360-0*   **$9.45**
*In the first place, Miss Minchin lived in London. Her home was a large, dull, tall one, in a large, dull square, where all the houses were alike, and all the
sparrows were alike, and where all the door-knockers made the same heavy sound...   Childrens/Classic Pages 88*

The Autobiography of Benjamin Franklin by *Benjamin Franklin*   ISBN: *1-59462-135-7*   **$24.95**
*The Autobiography of Benjamin Franklin has probably been more extensively read than any other American historical work, and no other book of its kind
has had such ups and downs of fortune. Franklin lived for many years in England, where he was agent...   Biographies/History Pages 332*

Name	
Email	
Telephone	
Address	
City, State ZIP	

☐ **Credit Card**   ☐ **Check / Money Order**

Credit Card Number	
Expiration Date	
Signature	

Please Mail to: Book Jungle
PO Box 2226
Champaign, IL 61825
or Fax to: 630-214-0564

ORDERING INFORMATION

web: *www.bookjungle.com*
email: *sales@bookjungle.com*
fax: *630-214-0564*
mail: *Book Jungle PO Box 2226 Champaign, IL 61825*
or PayPal *to sales@bookjungle.com*

Please contact us for bulk discounts

DIRECT-ORDER TERMS

**20% Discount if You Order
Two or More Books**
Free Domestic Shipping!
Accepted: Master Card, Visa,
Discover, American Express